Praise for
The Bipolar Workbook

"Dr. Basco once again hits it out of the park with this clear and concise workbook. This book can have a profound effect on improving the quality of life of anyone with bipolar illness."
—*Daniel J. Taylor, PhD, Department of Psychology, University of North Texas*

"Having suffered with bipolar disorder for years, I am grateful for Dr. Basco's well-organized, easy-to-understand guidance on how to live with this illness. The book contains numerous useful exercises that help you organize your thoughts in a logical way. It helps you understand your symptoms and moods and teaches realistic coping strategies so you can get your life back."
—*Erin B.*

"For those on the bipolar spectrum—as well as loved ones who want to understand and help—this book is empathic, respectful, empowering, and accessible. Dr. Basco's deep understanding of the illness is evident. The tools in this book can help you strengthen your commitment to treatment, practice essential coping skills, and achieve greater stability."
—*Cory F. Newman, PhD, ABPP, Center for Cognitive Therapy,*
Perelman School of Medicine, University of Pennsylvania

"This workbook successfully guides patients through the course of their illness at an easy-to-understand level and is specific to various stages of the illness. It will help patients gain awareness, understanding, knowledge, and ownership of their illness. . . . This is, undoubtedly, one of the best workbooks on bipolar disorder in a long time. It is thorough, realistic, and should be given to all bipolar patients as part of their treatment plan. Highly recommended! 5 stars!"
—Doody's Review Service

"A great book has gotten even better. The *Workbook* is an invaluable aide to managing bipolar disorder and achieving sustained wellness. I highly recommend this lucidly written book to people with bipolar illness and their families and friends."
—*Madhukar H. Trivedi, MD, Department of Psychiatry, University of Texas*
Southwestern Medical Center

"This workbook provides essential tools for coping with mood swings and intense emotions. Dr. Basco explains step by step how to manage the mix of depression and mania symptoms that typically goes along with bipolar disorder. A fantastic book and a 'must read.'"
—*Thilo Deckersbach, PhD, Department of Psychiatry,*
Massachusetts General Hospital and Harvard Medical School

"Extremely useful. . . . This is an excellent example of putting helpful, evidence-based tools and information in the hands of people . . . who are experiencing a baffling disorder."
—PsycCRITIQUES

The Bipolar Workbook

Also by Monica Ramirez Basco

Cognitive-Behavioral Therapy for Bipolar Disorder, Second Edition
Monica Ramirez Basco and A. John Rush

The Procrastinator's Guide to Getting Things Done
Monica Ramirez Basco

The Bipolar Workbook

Tools for Controlling Your Mood Swings

SECOND EDITION

Monica Ramirez Basco, PhD

THE GUILFORD PRESS
New York   London

© 2015 The Guilford Press
A Division of Guilford Publications, Inc.
370 Seventh Avenue, Suite 1200, New York, NY 10001
www.guilford.com

The information in this volume is not intended as a substitute for consultation with healthcare professionals. Each individual's health concerns should be evaluated by a qualified professional.

Printed in the United States of America

This book is printed on acid-free paper.

Last digit is print number: 9   8   7   6   5   4   3   2   1

Library of Congress Cataloging-in-Publication Data

Basco, Monica Ramirez.
    The bipolar workbook : tools for controlling your mood swings / Monica Ramirez Basco, PhD. — Second edition.
      pages   cm
    ISBN 978-1-4625-2023-7 (paperback)
    1. Manic–depressive illness—Popular works.   2. Manic–depressive illness—Treatment—Popular works.   3. Manic–depressive illness—Treatment—Problems, exercises, etc.   I. Title.
    RC516.B356 2015
    616.89'5—dc23
                                           2015001051

*To my husband, Michael—my best friend
and biggest fan—with all my love*

Contents

Step 4
Reduce Your Symptoms

Step 5
Strengthen Your Coping Skills

Purchasers can download and print select practical
tools from this book at *www.guilford.com/basco2-forms.*

Preface

Thank you for the opportunity to share with you this second edition of *The Bipolar Workbook: Tools for Controlling Your Mood Swings.* The first edition, which was published in 2006, was intended as a therapy supplement for people who were participating in cognitive-behavioral therapy for bipolar I disorder in addition to medication treatment. The exercises in the workbook included many that were commonly given as therapy homework. As it turned out, the workbook was used not only by people with bipolar I disorder, but also by clinicians, educators, family members, and people who suffered from mood swings of other types. It was translated into several languages, attesting to the fact that bipolar disorder is a problem that affects people all over the world.

Our understanding of bipolar disorder continues to grow as clinicians, scientists, and those who suffer from mood swings uncover new ways to address symptoms. Several new medications for mood disorders have become available since the publication of the first edition of this book, and we also know more about how people can play an active role in predicting, preventing, and controlling their mood episodes.

The exercises in the first edition of the workbook were tailored to those newly diagnosed with bipolar I disorder, those who had experience with the illness but had not yet achieved remission of symptoms, and those who had achieved control of their mood swings and were in a maintenance phase of treatment. We now know more about the many forms that mood symptoms can take even in people who receive the same diagnosis and how those symptoms can vary over time. It has also become clear that many people have mood swings that disrupt their lives even if their symptoms do not fit textbook definitions of depression and mania.

Therefore, this workbook is no longer organized around these three groups. Instead, the focus is on symptoms caused by a spectrum of disorders that share several common features. People who can benefit from this book have a pattern of episodes or periods during which symptoms start, reach a peak, and begin to taper off. This makes them predictable or, at least, possible to track. The mood swings seem to be triggered by things such as stress or seasons, so control of those triggers is a possibility. When mood swings occur, they affect how people think, act, and feel. They can interfere with normal functioning, and they can make people act in uncharacteristic ways.

The methods for catching and controlling mood swings that were included in the first edition have also been expanded to meet the needs of those who "feel bipolar" at times but do not necessarily have a diagnosis. In fact, most exercises are applicable to people who have normal types of moodiness or sometimes have difficulty coping with stress. More examples of symptoms, problems, life circumstances, and coping abilities have been added to the workbook through illustrations involving people whose mood swings range in severity from milder mood disorders to more severe forms of bipolar disorder.

To make the overall strategies for controlling your mood swings easier to follow, the chapters have been shortened and the exercises streamlined. Each chapter builds on the preceding one to help you move through the five steps to controlling your symptoms. You can skip through the sections that do not pertain to you or that cover skills you have already mastered.

What remains the same from the first edition is the goal of helping you learn new skills for identifying mood symptoms early in their development and use strategies for gaining control of those symptoms. The theoretical model that underlies the interventions is still cognitive-behavioral therapy, a well-tested and effective form of psychotherapeutic treatment. The hope is that this workbook will complement the strategies you are already using such as medication treatment and psychotherapy. So read ahead to get the big picture on your pattern of mood swings. Learn to see symptoms coming. Find out how to take quick action to avoid making matters worse, and to reduce your symptoms instead. And make it your goal to continually strengthen your coping skills so that you can take control of your mood swings.

The Bipolar Workbook

Step 1

Get the Big Picture

1

Understand How You Can Control Your Mood Swings

In this chapter you will:

- ✓ Find out what you can do to control your mood swings.
- ✓ Read about the five steps toward better control of your symptoms.
- ✓ Learn why medication may not be enough.
- ✓ Discover how this workbook can help.

Feeling Bipolar?

The word *bipolar* is usually used to describe a specific type of mood disorder in which people have severe mood swings called major depressive episodes and manic episodes. However, many people use the term *bipolar* to describe sudden or extreme shifts in mood, attitude, outlook, or behavior that cause problems in relationships or at work, lead to poor coping behaviors such as substance abuse, or result in poor decision making that leads to negative life consequences.

Mood shifts are normal human experiences. They can be reactions to positive or negative events such as successes or losses. They can occur in response to the words and actions of others. They can be driven by biological changes such as alterations in brain chemistry for people with psychiatric disorders, changes in blood sugar for those with diabetes, fluctuation in hormone levels, and physical illness or injury. Mood swings can also be the result of a combination of these forces acting at the same time.

If you have self-awareness, you might notice that you feel full of energy on some days and are tired or unmotivated on other days. **These fluctuations are considered normal unless they last too long, interfere with your ability to function normally, are accompanied by other physical and mental symptoms, or cause you a great deal of discomfort or distress.** Your mood swings may be noticeable to other people. You might have had the experience of friends or family members telling you that you are "acting bipolar," are "moody" or "unpredictable," have "multiple personalities," or just seem to be a different person depending on the day, the season, or the time of the month. This workbook is intended for people who suffer from these types of mood changes, and the goal is to become more aware of them and to gain as much control over them as possible.

Bipolar Spectrum Disorders

Bipolar I disorder is a psychiatric illness that affects about 1% of Americans. It generally starts in late adolescence or early adulthood and is lifelong once it begins. People who have bipolar I disorder usually experience periods of extreme depression that can last months at a time. They also experience periods of euphoria or extreme irritability that are called manic episodes. During manic episodes a person might have racing thoughts, feel a pressure to keep talking, be unable to sleep, and behave in ways that show poor judgment. Manic episodes can last anywhere from several weeks to several months. During this time, the person's ability to function worsens. Bipolar I disorder is one of the most severe and persistent mental illnesses.

There are other types of mood disorders that resemble bipolar disorder but are not as severe. They may not include experiences with mania, or may seem more like personality characteristics than an illness. Together, these are called bipolar spectrum disorders because they include people with a full range of symptoms on a spectrum from the most severe and chronic to those that share the features of bipolar disorder but occur infrequently and do not impair daily functioning. Chapter 2 will provide more information about these disorders.

While the first edition of this workbook focused specifically on bipolar I disorder, this second edition provides interventions for all types of mood swings on the bipolar spectrum. The exercises address symptoms of major depression and mania, but these strategies can also help to prevent or relieve the symptoms of hypomania, a milder form of mania, as well as mild depression, irritability, and anxiety.

What Can You Do about It?

There are many different strategies for controlling your mood swings. If you have a mood disorder such as bipolar I or bipolar II disorder, medication is a key to stabilizing your mood. If you are female and your mood swings are related to your menstrual cycle, your gynecologist may suggest hormones to even out your mood. If you have problems with your thyroid, poorly controlled diabetes, or another type of endocrine problem, your physician can work with you to try to resolve mood symptoms. If medical interventions are not enough or if your mood swings are not the result of a biological problem, you may be able to learn how to control your mood swings by making changes in your reactions, your attitudes, or your life situations.

Take Control of Your Mood

This workbook is designed to guide you through the process of learning what you can do, in addition to taking medication regularly, to control your mood swings. If you make the effort, you can learn to lessen and perhaps avoid severe mood swings as well as symptoms of depression, mania, hypomania, irritability, anger, and anxiety. You can also learn to cope with the many ways your mood symptoms interfere with your life. You can use this workbook on your own, make it part of your individual or group therapy, or work through it with your therapist or doctor. Each chapter offers information, skills, and exercises that can help you learn to cope with your emotions, control negative thinking, minimize physical symptoms, stick with medication treatment, and manage problems of daily life.

If you commit the time to practice and learn each method, this workbook can help you learn more about your mood swings, discover new ways to keep the symptoms from coming back, get more out of treatment, and work toward reaching your goals in life. To accomplish these things, you will need to learn how to do several important things:

1. Understand what is happening to you.
2. Recognize significant mood swings.
3. Not act in ways that make symptoms worse.
4. Reduce your symptoms by adjusting your actions, thoughts, and environment.
5. Strengthen yourself for the future by learning better ways to cope.

The chapters in this book are organized according to these goals. Below is a brief summary of what you can learn at each step. There are many different exercises throughout this workbook. Not all will apply to your unique situation and problems. Pick the ones that seem to suit you best. If they are not helpful, try some of the others.

GET THE BIG PICTURE

- Understand your mood swings and figure out what you can do to help yourself.
- Learn about the symptoms of bipolar disorder.
- Figure out the difference between a mood swing and the real you.

SEE IT COMING

- See the changes coming—learn to recognize and label your moods.
- Know what triggers your mood swings and improve your coping.

DON'T MAKE IT WORSE

- Avoid things that make your mood worse.
- Don't let emotions control your thinking.
- Stop avoidance and procrastination.

REDUCE YOUR SYMPTOMS

- Regain control when you feel overwhelmed.
- Change your negative outlook.
- Learn to analyze your thoughts.
- Work through denial about needing medication.
- Improve medication consistency.

STRENGTHEN YOUR COPING SKILLS

- Learn to deal effectively with problems.
- Strengthen your stress management skills and healthy habits.
- Make better decisions.
- Maintain your gains.

Why It Might Take More Than Medication

Medications that effectively control symptoms of depression and mania, mood swings, anxiety, irritability, and sleep problems are the cornerstone of managing severe mood swings like those common in bipolar disorder. Mood disorders are biological illnesses that cause changes in the way your brain processes the chemicals your body naturally produces. Medications are designed to correct this problem by providing these chemicals or neurotransmitters when they are lacking or by helping your brain use them more efficiently. Without medication, psychological approaches like those presented in this workbook may be only minimally effective for people who have severe mood swings. But even with medication, you may need more to gain the greatest possible control over your mood swings and to prevent relapses.

- You need backup interventions for those times when you don't take your medications consistently or when they are not working fully. Most people have trouble taking medication on a regular basis, especially when their symptoms have improved or when medication side effects are unpleasant.

- You need ways to minimize stress, cope with changes of season or life circumstances, and avoid sleep loss—all factors that can cause symptoms to return even when you take medication every day.

- You need healthy and effective ways to control your symptoms instead of giving in to the temptation to use alcohol or street drugs to help you sleep, calm your anxiety, or change your mood. Alcohol and street drugs are not safe to use when you are taking psychiatric medications, they can interfere with the potency of some medications, and they can make your mood swings worse.

• You need methods for examining and managing your lifestyle so that it doesn't lead to sleep loss, poor eating habits, or unhealthy behaviors that can increase the risk of relapse.

• You need some strategies for sorting out your feelings about your mood swings and treatment when you feel conflicted about it. You may find yourself going through times when part of you rejects the idea of having to take medications to control your mood or is unwilling to make the modifications to your lifestyle that might help reduce or eliminate symptoms. At the same time another part of you knows what you should do to take care of yourself.

• You need ways to reverse the mental meltdown that makes it hard to think. Mood swings can make it hard to organize your thoughts, make decisions, and solve problems.

• You need ways to resolve the problems that stress you so that you can improve the quality of your life. Medications may remove symptoms, but if you've had financial, legal, or family problems as a result of your symptoms, you'll be left with those problems even when your mood swings have improved.

Fortunately, there are methods you can learn to fill the gaps that medication treatment leaves. Strategies for controlling symptoms, preventing relapse, and solving problems are explained in this workbook. Mastering these strategies will help you come to terms with your illness, give you a reason to stick with medication treatment, and keep the ups and downs from interfering with your life.

How Does It Work?

Many different things can trigger mood swings. They can include reactions to upsetting or exciting events, a stressful interaction with a significant other, important news—either good or bad, lack of sleep, hunger, physical illness, or concern for other people. In people who have mood disorders, shifts into mania or depression can be triggered by taking medications inconsistently or not at all, changes in seasons, illness, or trauma, or they can occur for no obvious reason at all. Once a mood swing starts, however, your reaction to it can make symptoms better or worse. A goal of this workbook is to help you recognize mood shifts, pause long enough to think through your choices of action, and handle the situation in a way that is helpful and not hurtful to you in the long run. Here are some examples, which are composites designed to represent experiences common among those struggling with mood problems.

Tommy is a struggling college student. He has had two episodes of mania so far. The first episode was mild and did not last very long. He was diagnosed with bipolar disorder after his second episode because his symptoms were bad enough to require hospitalization. The police took him to the emergency room when he crashed his car into a light pole. It took several hospitalizations before Tommy began to feel like his old self. Throughout the workbook, examples of Tommy's efforts to work through the exercises will be provided.

Like most people who have been newly diagnosed, Tommy knew very little about bipolar disorder, but he was pretty certain that he did not have it. He picked up the book from time to time and read through sections that caught his eye but did not really work through the entire program right away. His psychiatrist encouraged him to read more and learn about what he could do to control his symptoms. Tommy read the first few chapters, about the illness, but was not ready to buy into the idea that he had bipolar disorder. His mom was very worried about Tommy and frustrated by his lack of effort to educate himself. She read through the workbook as well as many other books on bipolar disorder so she would understand what was happening to her son. Eventually, Tommy began to use the workbook like a reference book. Each time he had a new experience that might be related to bipolar disorder, he tried to find an exercise related to it.

Amanda is a good example of someone who has dealt with the many ups and downs of bipolar disorder but does not feel confident that she can control it. She is a 32-year-old nurse who had her first episode of major depression in high school and her first manic episode in nursing school about 6 years ago. She has had other periods of depression, mania, and hypomania and has been under the care of a psychiatrist off and on over many years. In addition, Amanda has had supportive counseling and attends a self-help group to cope with periods of low mood. She knows she has bipolar disorder and wants to do what she can to control it for the sake of her family. She suffers from low-level depression much of the time and often has difficulty keeping her home clean and organized, doing her job at the hospital, and caring for her 5-year-old daughter and 12-year-old son. She has lost jobs for poor attendance when she was depressed and has walked off of jobs because her irritability and impulsiveness during manic spells have gotten the best of her.

Amanda picked up this workbook after a period of depression that really frightened her. She caught herself thinking that life was not worth living and that there was no hope for a better future. This was not Amanda's usual attitude, and when she came out of the depression, it greatly upset her that she had allowed her thinking to get so distorted. She kept thinking, "What if I had acted on those ideas?" Amanda was ready to work diligently through all the exercises in the workbook. She recognized her symptoms from the examples in Chapters 2 and 3 and knew she had coped poorly with them in the past. Amanda was particularly interested in learning to control her distorted thinking, so she slowly and carefully worked through each exercise in Chapters 7, 10, and 11. Amanda's examples are included throughout the workbook. If you think you're like Amanda, pay particular attention to how she completed each exercise.

Paul and Raquel are both good examples of people who have learned a great deal about how to manage bipolar disorder. Both have had bad experiences with depression and did not want to go there again. Paul is 24 years old, but his bipolar disorder started during his elementary school years and he has been through enough treatment to be an expert on the issue. He is a software engineer working for a small start-up company. He spends most of his time building websites for other companies, but he has a number of creative ideas and plans to start his own company before he turns 30. Paul did not go through a period of denial like Tommy had, because his parents explained to him when he was a young child what illness he had and how medication would help. He learned early in life that he felt better with medication than without it and that things went better at school and with his friends when he was more stable. Although Paul knew a great deal about the biology of bipolar disorder and was pretty consistent with taking medications, he did not know much about how his reactions contributed to his symptoms. He wanted to learn what he could do to keep his symptoms from flaring up without always having to take additional medications, which had been his strategy in the past. Paul only skimmed through the first three chapters because he had already read so much about the illness, as had his parents. What he wanted to learn were the methods in Chapters 5 and 6 for making himself less vulnerable to relapse by controlling his actions. Although he knew himself pretty well, he did not always recognize symptoms until they were severe and easily noticeable to others. Examples of how Paul worked through each exercise are provided throughout the workbook.

Raquel is 45 years old and has found a medication regimen that works well for her. She rarely has severe symptoms, and when they do occur she makes adjustments in her medication and in her actions to control them. She does a very good job of holding off the emergence of mania, but she still can become overwhelmed by stress, which usually leads to depression. She has struggled with low self-esteem much of her life, and when things go wrong she has a tendency to blame herself, feel hopeless, and cope by overeating. She wanted to learn how to control what she thought were overreactions to stress. What appealed most to Raquel were the sections in the workbook that focused more on the symptoms of depression. Like Amanda, she had a problem with negative thinking not only when she was depressed, but also when her stress level was high. Raquel put more effort into the exercises in Chapters 7, 10, and 11 than into the others. She was amazed to find out in Chapter 6 how many things she had been doing that probably worsened her depression. She also learned how to add positive experiences to her life and how to climb out of the rut of lethargy and procrastination. Her responses to the exercises are provided throughout to give you an idea of how Raquel learned to control her reactions to stress.

Raquel has an older brother, Stan, who also has bipolar disorder. His has always been more severe. When he is manic, he experiences psychotic symptoms, like hearing voices and feeling paranoid. A few examples have been provided of how Stan has learned to cope with some of his symptoms.

Miguel has bipolar II disorder with more depression than hypomania. He had a drinking problem in his early 20s that is now pretty much under control. He is almost 40 and is married to Desiree. He read through Chapters 2 and 3, but he is not convinced that he has bipolar disorder. He recognized the symptoms of depression described in Chapters 8 and 10, but he thinks his hypomanic symptoms are the real him. He wasn't interested in reading Chapter 12 on denial, but his wife found it very helpful in understanding why bipolar disorder is hard for Miguel to accept. Miguel and Desiree have marital problems caused by his hypomanic behavior and her unwillingness to talk about their problems. They used the exercise in Chapter 8 to help them stop avoiding the issue.

Maria is a 30-year-old woman. She is gay, but her parents do not know it. She has bipolar I disorder but suffers primarily from depression. Her mood-stabilizing medications keep her manic symptoms under control. Maria's family has not accepted her illness. They put demands on her even when she is feeling bad, and because she feels guilty about being gay, she does everything she can to avoid disappointing her parents. Maria needs help with self-criticism when she is depressed, so she has focused her attention on the chapters that help her control her negative thoughts. She pushes herself even when she is feeling low or stressed out. The stress management strategies in Chapter 15 are helping her manage her stress and reduce her depression.

Joe has bipolar II disorder. Like Miguel, he has also struggled with alcohol problems through much of his adult life. Joe's wife Sarah found this workbook and asked him to read it. He isn't always aware of his mood swings, and Sarah thought he should learn more about them. Sarah's hope is that Joe will never have another major mood episode and will stay sober for the rest of this life. Joe tries to stay optimistic and tells Sarah that he has his illness under control, but he worries about it too. Joe made a commitment to Sarah that he would try to become more aware of when he is hypomanic, so he put extra effort into the exercises in Chapters 4, 5, and 6.

What's Next?

The purpose of this chapter was to introduce you to strategies in this workbook that can help you control symptoms of major depression, mania, and other less severe mood swings. The five steps for better control of your mood swings will be described in greater detail in the following chapters along with exercises that will help you put the ideas into action. Throughout the workbook you will be able to see how the people described in this chapter used the various exercises and activities to help control their symptoms.

In the next chapter you will learn more about the specific symptoms of depression and mania, the diagnosis of bipolar disorder, and the challenges to making an accurate diagnosis. You will be introduced to exercises intended to help you make personal use of the material presented.

2

Learn about the Symptoms of Bipolar Disorder

In this chapter you will:

✓ Discover the difference between having bipolar disorder and having mood swings.

✓ Find out how a diagnosis of bipolar disorder is made.

✓ Learn about common symptoms of depression, mania, and mixed episodes.

This chapter offers some basic information about bipolar disorder, including its diagnosis and related disorders. This description of the disorder does not replace a thorough evaluation by a trained clinician, but it will give you an idea of how doctors go about deciding whether or not you have bipolar disorder.

The *Diagnostic and Statistical Manual of Mental Disorders* (DSM-5), published by the American Psychiatric Association in 2013, provides guidelines for diagnosing mental illnesses. The DSM provides a description of the common features of each diagnosis, including how the symptoms might differ in children and adults, men and women, and people from different cultures. It provides diagnostic rules that describe the types and number of symptoms required to make a diagnosis and some rules for how long those symptoms must exist before a diagnosis can be made.

For all psychiatric disorders, the specific symptoms have to occur together in time. For example, if your symptoms of mania included rapid speech, hyperactivity, and a euphoric mood, these symptoms would have to occur at the same time and last for a while before they could be considered a disorder. This rule is intended to keep clinicians from overdiagnosing things that everyone experiences from time to time. For example, some people normally talk fast. So talking fast would not necessarily be a symptom. Hyperactivity is also a matter of opinion. If you are easygoing and accustomed to low levels of noise and activity, someone who is highly energetic and raring to go might strike you as hyperactive instead of as just more hyper than you. And anyone can feel euphoric for short periods of time, especially when experiencing good things.

Some indicators that you may be having symptoms that are "clinically significant"— those that a clinician would consider important—are that they:

- Occur together in time.
- Differ from your normal self.
- Cannot be explained away by a specific event or circumstance.
- Persist for several days to several weeks.
- Have started to cause you some problems.

Making a correct diagnosis of bipolar disorder is like putting together a puzzle. After pieces of information are gathered and assembled, the clinician looks for patterns. To gather clues, a clinician might ask about changes in your mood, behavior, and thoughts. He or she would also be interested in your functioning at home and work, any new problems you've had, any illnesses that could have caused your symptoms, and your use of alcohol and street drugs. Clinicians will also want to know something about what you were like before the symptoms began. It is especially helpful at this point if family members or friends can share their observations about what you used to be like and how you have changed. If the clinician suspects that you have a medical problem unrelated to bipolar disorder that may be causing your symptoms, you might be asked to undergo some laboratory tests, such as a blood test. You can also expect questions about the psychiatric history of your family members. Mood disorders run in families. So if your mother had a mood disorder and an uncle had one, there is a chance that you have one too. Finally, an experienced clinician who is familiar with bipolar disorder will make observations about what he or she sees in your mood, your behavior, your speech pattern, and your thought processes. With this information in hand, the clinician will review the diagnostic guidelines for bipolar disorder in DSM-5 to see if you meet the criteria.

What Is Mania?

To be diagnosed with bipolar disorder, DSM-5 says you must have had **at least one manic episode**. A manic episode is the experience of a high, euphoric, or overly irritable mood that lasts at least 1 week or requires hospitalization to control it. At the same time, you must have three or four of the other symptoms described in the section below. You have to have several symptoms at the same time so the clinician can be certain that this is really a clinically significant problem. Each symptom is something that many people experience even if they do not have bipolar disorder. The reason that four symptoms are required if you have an irritable rather than an expansive or elevated mood is that people get irritable, have trouble sleeping, and have poor concentration when they are depressed too. Requiring four symptoms helps clinicians be more certain that what is happening is actually a manic episode.

Read about each symptom of mania and make a note about the ones you have experienced. When you have finished this section, fill in Exercise 2.1 on page 17 to tally up how many symptoms of mania you have experienced.

High, euphoric, or overly irritable mood that lasts at least 1 week or requires hospitalization to control it

Euphoria is more than just a very good mood. It is feeling on top of the world, as if you couldn't possibly feel better, or feeling high as if on drugs without having taken any. Sometimes with mania, your mood can be so irritable that you argue with people, get into fights, or can't stand the feel of your own skin. A key sign of mania is when your mood swings into euphoria or irritability; it is different from your normal mood and it lasts all day for several days or weeks. It is not just a reaction to events in your life. For a diagnosis of mania, you must have this symptom and three to four of the others that follow.

Euphoric or irritable mood

☐ I think that I have had this symptom.

What did it feel like?

Unrealistic positive self-view

Inflated self-esteem is not the same as just feeling good about yourself, acting arrogant, or being full of yourself. This symptom is a positive self-view that goes beyond what would be considered normal for you or for most people. You might find yourself thinking that you're far superior to or incredibly more attractive than anyone you know. Or you might think that your ideas are the most brilliant ever, that they have no flaws, and that you're destined to get rich as a result. These claims could, of course, be true, but if you normally have much lower self-esteem or there is nothing to back up your claim, feeling this way might be considered a symptom. Grandiosity is a positive view taken to such a high level that you cannot see what is real and what is not.

Unrealistic positive self-view

☐ I think that I have had this symptom.

What did it feel like?

Feeling like you don't need much sleep or can get along with little sleep

If you have this symptom, you may find yourself feeling rested even though you are sleeping less than usual at night. You may have trouble getting to sleep, sleep fewer hours than is normal for you, or wake up much earlier than usual. If you usually get 7 to 8 hours of sleep, that amount might be reduced to 4 or 5 hours, or you may be unable to sleep at all. What makes it a symptom of mania is that you seem to have enough energy to make it through the day even though you are sleeping less. In this sense, it's different from the insomnia people experience when stressed or depressed. In those cases less sleep leaves people feeling exhausted. In mania, sometimes people do not feel the need to sleep until they have gone several days without it.

Feeling like you don't need much sleep

☐ I think that I have had this symptom.

What did it feel like?

Unusually talkative or feeling compelled to keep talking

This symptom tends to be more noticeable to others than to the person who has it. You may not feel like you're talking fast. In fact, it may seem to you that others are talking more slowly than usual. What you might notice is that you are tripping over your words or feeling tongue-tied because you're going too fast. You might even feel pressured to keep talking. What may be more noticeable are the comments from others that you're talking too much, jumping from subject to subject, or interrupting others when they are trying to take their turn to talk.

Unusually talkative or feeling compelled to keep talking

☐ I think that I have had this symptom.

What did it feel like?

Thoughts or ideas race through your mind at high speed

When racing thoughts are mild, it may seem like you just have more ideas or more thoughts running through your mind. The thoughts might seem at first to be more insightful or creative than usual, like you really understand things that other people miss. As this symptom progresses, you may find it hard to concentrate. Many people complain that they lose the ability to hold their thoughts together when they are manic. They lose their train of thought too quickly and feel frustrated by this. They can also have trouble getting their ideas across to others. At their most extreme, racing thoughts can seem like they are going too fast to be expressed aloud. They stop making sense to you and may no longer seem creative or brilliant. They bombard your mind, making it hard to have a conversation or even to fall asleep at night. You might want to turn them off, like turning off a radio, but you can't easily make them stop.

Speedy or racing thoughts

☐ I think that I have had this symptom.

What did it feel like?

More easily distracted than usual

Distractibility is an annoying symptom of mania that interferes with concentration, decision making, organization, and task completion. When this symptom occurs, you may find yourself distracted by external stimuli, like noise, lights, people, or activities going on around you. This might feel irritating to you or make you anxious. You might also be distracted by internal thoughts such as new ideas, memories, or urges to engage in new activities. Others may notice that you seem to start projects but get distracted and do not finish them.

Easily distracted

☐ I think that I have had this symptom.

What did it feel like?

Extreme restlessness or hyperactivity

Fueled by an increased number of ideas and greater energy than usual, many people find they are more physically active when manic. If you've previously gone through an episode of depression during which you got behind on chores or other responsibilities, the extra energy and motivation that come at the beginning of mania can be highly welcomed. You feel the urge to do more and have the energy to do it. Problems come when racing thoughts and distractibility keep you from completing the tasks you've started or when impaired judgment leads you to take action in ways that could cause you problems down the line or be more than you can handle.

Psychomotor agitation is another symptom of mania. It is not directed toward a goal. It is restlessness or an excess of nervous energy. You may have difficulty or feel uncomfortable and irritated when having to sit still. This restless feeling can appear at first as small repetitive movements like tapping your foot or biting your nails, but it usually progresses to pacing, rocking, or other kinds of action that help burn off some of this excessive nervous energy.

Extreme restlessness or hyperactivity

☐ I think that I have had this symptom.

What did it feel like?

Risk-taking

Risk-taking includes spending sprees, sexual indiscretions, and driving too fast or taking more risks on the road than is normal for you. This is more than just being adventurous by nature. Risk-taking can and often does lead to significant consequences for you or others. In fact, this is the symptom that catches the attention of family, friends, police officers, or health care providers and is the one that often leads to being evaluated for a psychiatric illness.

Risk-taking

☐ I think that I have had this symptom.

What did it feel like?

If manic symptoms are severe enough to require hospitalization, it's usually because you're too sick to take medications on your own, you're suicidal, you're too impaired to take care of your own basic needs, you can't fall asleep and as a result are becoming physically ill, you have forgotten to eat and are malnourished, or you are highly irritable and are making threats to harm others. Usually, if you have had mania before, you might become aware that you can't manage at home alone, you need medication to induce sleep, or you're not clear-minded enough to handle your medications, or you might fear doing something stupid or

EXERCISE 2.1 Which Symptoms of Mania Have You Experienced?

Place a check (✓) next to each symptom you have experienced. Circle the ones that have caused problems or interfered with your life.

Symptom of mania

☐ Euphoric or irritable mood

☐ Unrealistic positive self-view

☐ Feeling like you don't need much sleep

☐ Unusually talkative or feeling compelled to keep talking

☐ Speedy or racing thoughts

☐ Easily distracted

☐ Extreme restlessness or hyperactivity

☐ Risk-taking

_____ **Total number of symptoms experienced**

---

dangerous and causing harm to yourself or to others. In those cases you might request hospitalization yourself. However, more often it is family or friends who recognize the severity of the symptoms and call for help.

If you had the symptoms of mania, but they were caused by a medical problem, a medication, or substances of abuse, you would be diagnosed with what is called a *mood disorder due to a general medical condition* or a *mood disorder due to substance abuse*. This would not be considered a true manic episode. If this was the only time you were manic, you would not qualify for a diagnosis of bipolar disorder. However, it is not uncommon for a person to have had a true manic episode at one time in life and a manic episode that was due to a general medical condition at another time in life. When this is the case, the diagnosis stands as bipolar disorder, but the treatment would involve resolution of the general medical condition and not just treatment of the symptoms of mania.

- *Medical conditions* that can cause manic-like symptoms include degenerative neurological diseases such as Huntington's disease or multiple sclerosis, strokes, vitamin deficiencies, hyperthyroidism, infections, and some cancers.
- *Substances of abuse* that can cause manic-like symptoms include alcohol, amphetamines, cocaine, hallucinogens, inhalants, opioids, sedatives, hypnotics, and anxiolytics.

- *Medications* that can cause manic-like symptoms include antidepressant medications of all types, corticosteroids, anabolic steroids, antiparkinson medications, and some decongestants.

What Is Major Depression?

Most people who have bipolar disorder have suffered through episodes of depression as well as mania. There are many types of depression, but the one that people with bipolar disorder have is called *major depression.* Clinicians usually refer to major depression in people who have bipolar disorder as *bipolar depression*; they call it *unipolar depression* in people who have never had mania or hypomania. *Unipolar* means one end or direction. This means you feel the lows of major depression but never have the highs of mania. *Bipolar* means two ends or directions—up and down. This means you have experienced the highs of mania at some point in your life as well as the lows of major depression.

Read about the symptoms of major depression in the following pages and make a note about the ones you have experienced in Exercise 2.2 on page 23. Keep in mind that a diagnosis of major depression requires five or more symptoms during the same 2-week period. One of the five symptoms must be either depressed mood or loss of interest or pleasure in your usual activities. Five or more symptoms are required because each individual symptom of major depression is something that many people experience from time to time even when they are not depressed. To be certain that the symptoms are indicative of major depression, lots of them have to be present together. The reason that symptoms must last for at least 2 weeks before they are considered clinically important is to keep clinicians from making the mistake of diagnosing depression when it may be only a normal reaction to stress, moodiness caused by hormone fluctuations, or symptoms caused by a brief medical illness.

The symptoms of depression must be bothersome or interfere with your usual level of functioning to be considered clinically significant. This criterion is sometimes difficult to meet in people whose usual level of functioning is quite high. Impairment brings them down to a lower level but still leaves them in good enough shape to make it through each day. In this case, the criterion is satisfied when people are greatly troubled by the symptoms or the extra effort to cope is beginning to wear them out or they find themselves losing their ability to "fake it."

Low or sad mood

When depressed, some people feel sad and are tearful, the way they might feel if they were grieving. Others feel empty or lonely, or may feel a lack of emotion. It's not unusual for a depressed mood to be mixed with irritability, anger, or anxiety. For the most severe forms of depression, the sad mood does not improve even when good things happen. Those who experience this level of sadness say they understand that they should be happy, but they don't feel anything. In some types of depression, mood improves when pleasant or positive things happen such as during a celebration, when hearing good news, or when a loved one visits. This is called a *reactive mood.* Unfortunately, the person's mood quickly returns to depression when the event is over.

> **Low or sad mood**
>
> ☐ I think that I have had this symptom.
>
> What did it feel like?

Loss of interest and little enjoyment

When clinicians ask people if they have lost interest or pleasure in their usual activities, most depressed people say they have not had the energy to do anything enjoyable or interesting in some time. That makes it hard for them to know whether they have lost interest or are just too tired or unmotivated to take part in activities. Loss of interest or enjoyment is not limited to big events like vacations or parties. It's usually noticeable during everyday events and includes enjoying work less than usual and not wanting to play with the kids, visit with friends, or spend time on hobbies. It also includes avoiding phone calls from friends, not reading as much as usual, not really wanting to hear about other people's activities, and taking little or no pleasure in eating, watching television, or going to movies. It's important to distinguish loss of interest and enjoyment from loss of energy. When it is an interest and pleasure problem, there is no desire to participate in activities, even when you have the energy to do so.

> **Loss of interest and little enjoyment**
>
> ☐ I think that I have had this symptom.
>
> What did it feel like?

Unusual changes in appetite and/or weight

When depressed, some people have no interest in food. They may not feel hungry, or they may just have trouble deciding what to eat. Even with no appetite, people often eat anyway, especially comfort foods, sweets, or soft foods that take little effort to eat. This symptom also includes getting less enjoyment from food or loss of taste for your usual favorites. Eating less usually results in weight loss. Some people have a surge in their appetite when depressed and find themselves eating even when not hungry. This often leads to weight gain.

Unusual changes in appetite and/or weight

☐ I think that I have had this symptom.

What did it feel like?

Trouble with falling or staying asleep or sleeping too much

There are many ways that your sleep can be disturbed. One is called *initial insomnia,* which occurs when you have more trouble falling asleep than is normal for you (most people normally fall asleep in less than 30 minutes). Initial insomnia is so frustrating that some people deal with it by not going to bed until they are extremely exhausted or by engaging in some other activity like watching television or surfing the Internet until they feel tired enough to fall asleep. *Middle insomnia* occurs when you wake up several times during the night. The sleep you do get is fitful and not restful, and you awake feeling tired. Waking up to use the bathroom, get a drink of water, or check on a noise that woke you is not insomnia if you can go back to sleep quickly. A third type of insomnia is called *terminal insomnia.* This occurs when you wake up an hour or more earlier than you intend and can't go back to sleep.

Hypersomnia is the opposite problem, sleeping much more than normal because you go to bed a lot earlier than usual or take naps during the day, or feel sleepy throughout the day despite getting enough sleep. With hypersomnia, sleep is usually fairly sound but causes problems because you're sleeping rather than engaging in other activities such as interacting with others, doing chores, or having fun.

Trouble with falling or staying asleep or sleeping too much

☐ I think that I have had this symptom.

What did it feel like?

Feeling restless or slowed down

Psychomotor agitation includes restlessness, pacing, and generally having difficulty sitting still for long periods of time. You might find yourself getting up and walking around at work more often than usual, having trouble sitting through a movie, or preferring movement to inactivity despite being tired. If you don't give in to the urge to move around, you may feel irritable, lose your focus or concentration, or find that you can't stand the feel of your own skin.

Feeling restless or slowed down

☐ I think that I have had this symptom.

What did it feel like?

Exhaustion

Loss of energy is one of the first things that people notice when they are getting depressed. They tire more easily than usual, running out of steam to complete normal activities. Even after getting enough sleep, depression can make you feel tired, but if coupled with insomnia, the low energy is worse. As mentioned earlier, in the section on loss of interest and enjoyment, it is easy to confuse lack of motivation and lack of energy. You can have the desire but lack the physical energy to engage in your normal routine. People who have this symptom say that they want to clean their house, wash their car, or buy groceries, but they don't have enough energy to do it on their own.

Exhaustion

☐ I think that I have had this symptom.

What did it feel like?

Feeling worthless or guilty

Some people are always hard on themselves or have low self-esteem. This is not the same thing as feelings of worthlessness. Worthlessness is when you feel you have little value as a human being or that your existence is meaningless. This is much worse than low self-esteem or self-criticism. People with this symptom feel unworthy or unlovable, and encouragement from others does not change their minds. Excessive guilt can contribute to feelings of worthlessness if you blame yourself for things that are not your fault or find it impossible to forgive yourself for your mistakes.

Feeling worthless or guilty

☐ I think that I have had this symptom.

What did it feel like?

Poor concentration or trouble with making decisions

Those who suffer from poor concentration and indecisiveness find it difficult to read or follow the story line of a movie or television show. You may find yourself having to reread paragraphs of an article or a story because you keep losing your place.

It is not only the big decisions that can be hard to make when you're depressed. You might also find that smaller decisions about what to wear, what to eat, or what to do first can also seem more complicated, difficult, or burdensome than usual. For example, you stare into the refrigerator for long periods of time because you can't decide what to eat. You stand in front of your open closet and can't decide what to wear. You repeatedly flip through television channels but can't find anything that looks interesting. It can feel like there are too many choices and too many decisions to make and you would be happier if someone would just make a few for you.

Poor concentration or trouble with making decisions

☐ I think that I have had this symptom.

What did it feel like?

Suicidal thoughts

When depression is severe and nothing seems to make it better, people think about death as an alternative. They are in emotional pain and believe that one way to relieve the pain is to no longer exist. This is a dangerous fantasy. Sometimes these thoughts involve a specific plan to kill oneself and ideas about when to do so. More often, however, suicidal thoughts are more vague or general. No plan has been made, and the person is pretty certain that he or she will not do it, but thinking about the possibility brings some peace, as if it means there is a way out of the discomfort. Other forms this symptom takes include a desire to disappear, to fall asleep and never wake up, or to contract an incurable illness that will take you quickly. A milder form involves not caring if you live or die or believing that life is not worth living.

Suicidal thoughts

☐ I think that I have had this symptom.

What did it feel like?

As with any other psychiatric illness, it's important not to confuse major depression with symptoms caused by some other biological process such as a general medical condition or illness, treatment for it, or a side effect of substance abuse.

- *Medical conditions* that can be mistaken for depression include neurological illnesses such as Parkinson's disease, stroke, vitamin deficiencies, endocrine problems such as hypothyroidism, infections, hepatitis, mononucleosis, or cancer.
- *Substances of abuse* that can cause symptoms of depression include alcohol, amphetamines, cocaine, hallucinogens, opioids, sedatives, or inhalants.
- *Medications* such as antihypertensives, oral contraceptives, anabolic steroids, anti-cancer agents, analgesics, and cardiac medications can also produce depression-like symptoms.

EXERCISE 2.2   ## Which Symptoms of Major Depression Have You Experienced?

Place a check (✓) next to each symptom you have experienced. Circle the ones that have caused problems or interfered with your life.

Symptom of depression

☐ Low or sad mood

☐ Loss of interest and little enjoyment

☐ Unusual changes in appetite and/or weight

☐ Trouble with falling or staying asleep or sleeping too much

☐ Restless or slowed down

☐ Exhaustion

☐ Feeling worthless or guilty

☐ Poor concentration or trouble with making decisions

☐ Suicidal thoughts

_____ **Total number of symptoms experienced**

Why It's Hard to Make a Diagnosis of Bipolar Disorder

There are two big challenges in making a diagnosis of bipolar disorder, each of which can lead to error and interfere with treatment. The first challenge is timing, and the second is accuracy.

Timing

Bipolar disorder can look different depending on when in the course of the illness a diagnosis is made. People with bipolar disorder will be in different states across the course of their lives. There will be periods of depression, periods of mania, and periods of wellness. The periods of illness are called *episodes*. An episode starts with mild symptoms, reaches a peak of severity in the symptoms, and then begins to improve. Therefore, the accuracy of a diagnosis will depend on the clarity and severity of the symptoms. For example, if you were having a major depressive episode, you would look a little tired and a little blue at the beginning of the episode but eventually reach a low point, called the *nadir*, when the symptoms are at their worst. At the nadir, you might have severe insomnia, be too tired to go to work, feel so hopeless that life does not seem worth living, and find that you no longer care about yourself or others. It would not be unusual at the nadir of an episode to hear voices that others cannot hear, to have your eyes play tricks on you to the degree that you see things that other people cannot see, or to become convinced that people are trying to hurt you when there is no real evidence that this is the case. These are called *psychotic symptoms*. They occur when depression is at its worst, but they also occur in psychotic disorders such as schizophrenia or schizoaffective disorder. If a clinician saw you when you were at your worst and having psychotic symptoms, you might be diagnosed inaccurately as having one of these disorders instead of bipolar disorder.

If you were seen toward the end of an episode of depression, you would look like you did at the beginning of the episode, with milder symptoms, able to function fairly well, but perhaps not yet feeling happy. If you were seen between episodes, when you were no longer having major depression or mania, you would look fine. No one would suspect that you have a mental illness.

The same course applies to mania. At the beginning you would probably look a little hyper, be a little more talkative, and have more self-confidence than usual. It might look like an improvement if you had previously been through an episode of depression. As the symptoms of mania progress and reach their peak you might become agitated, irritable, unable to sit still, and difficult to understand, and you would likely be exercising poor judgment in some way. You might also be grandiose, thinking that you have special powers or that you are more intelligent or gifted than anyone else. At this peak, you might also hear voices telling you to take chances, and you might see visions that you believe are real and have special meaning for you, such as seeing God or angels. These are also *psychotic symptoms*. If you came into an emergency room talking about your visions and the voices you were hearing and unable to tell about your history of depression and mania, you would very likely be mistaken as having a psychotic disorder like schizophrenia or schizoaffective disorder. If you had also been using street drugs or drinking alcohol, someone might think your symptoms were just a sign of a severe substance abuse problem.

Some people come down from the high of mania and plunge into an episode of depression rather than returning to their normal self. An episode of mania can leave you feeling exhausted, out of sorts, disoriented, and unable to function well on your own. If you were seen at this point and your history was not apparent, it might be hard to know whether you were ending a mania or in the middle of a depression.

Another complexity related to timing is the age at which the symptoms began. In adults, mania and depression are fairly easy to distinguish from normal states. Manias are often euphoric, and the person feels better than good. Depressions make people feel sad or tearful. When bipolar disorder begins in childhood or during adolescence, the picture is not as clear. Kids are more likely to feel irritable and angry than sad or euphoric. Also, kids are not as able as adults to verbalize feeling states. They know that they feel bad, but they may not be able to be more specific. Children do not have the coping abilities of adults, so when they feel bad they may act up in ways that look like misbehavior. They may be argumentative, defiant, uncompromising, and impulsive in much the same way that kids do who have conduct disorder problems, hyperactivity, or attention deficit disorder. If you were diagnosed early in life, it is likely that you would be given one of these more common childhood diagnoses and treated accordingly.

Another timing concern is in the progression of the illness. Suppose that in the early phases of your illness you had two episodes of major depression before you ever had your first manic episode. Let's say the first episode occurred at the age of 16, when your parents divorced. You may have gotten some therapy, or it may have passed on its own, but it would not have been accurate to diagnose you with bipolar disorder after just one episode of depression. The correct diagnosis would have been *major depression.*

If you had another episode of depression when you finished high school and were heading to college or your first job, most people would have said that it was just stress because you were not sure where you were going in life or were afraid to be on your own. You probably would have not sought treatment unless the symptoms caused you to drop out of school or lose your job. At that point, the correct diagnosis for you would have been *recurrent major depression.* However, if, like many people, you had figured out that alcohol or street drugs made you feel better temporarily when depressed, the diagnostic picture would have been even more confusing. When depression and alcohol or substance abuse occur at the same time, it is very difficult to tell which caused which. When you had your first manic episode, however, your diagnosis would have been changed from recurrent major depression to *bipolar disorder.*

In this example, the correct diagnosis changed as the illness progressed. The initial diagnosis of major depression would have been correct because mania had not yet occurred and no one could have known that it was coming. The fact that the diagnosis was changed to bipolar disorder after mania happened for the first time does not mean that the first diagnosis of major depression was wrong. It was correct at the time it was given. After a diagnosis of bipolar disorder is given, the old diagnosis of recurrent major depression no longer applies. Instead, the diagnosis of bipolar disorder becomes your primary diagnosis. Doctors understand that when you have bipolar disorder you will have periods of depression as well as periods of mania, hypomania, and mixed states.

The point of explaining how these complications can interfere with a correct diagnosis is to help you understand how the diagnostic process can be challenging. If you think that the timing of your symptoms might have led clinicians to draw the wrong conclusion about you, ask your doctor to explain why he or she thinks you have bipolar disorder or get another clinical opinion on your diagnosis. Rather than reject a diagnosis, get more information about it.

Accuracy

Research studies on the accuracy of diagnoses made by clinicians consistently show that errors can be made. Despite advances in other areas of medicine, psychiatry, which deals with the most complex organ, the brain, does not yet have the technology to accurately detect physical indicators of specific illnesses such as bipolar disorder. Because there are no current laboratory tests that can confirm the existence of mental illnesses in individuals, all diagnoses are made by reviewing the person's symptoms and determining whether the pattern meets the DSM-5 criteria discussed in this chapter. Making a correct judgment depends on the amount of information available to the clinician as well as the thoroughness of the clinician and his or her level of training and skill. With so many variables at work, there is a lot of room for error.

Mistakes in diagnosis are made most often for two reasons: (1) the patient is not able to provide enough information on his or her history and progression of symptoms to aid diagnosis, and (2) several different psychological or medical problems may be occurring simultaneously, such as depression and alcohol use or mania and cocaine use or mood symptoms and psychotic symptoms. Adding to the complexity of the picture are cultural and geographic differences in the way symptoms appear and the words used to describe them. For example, what looks like hypomania in West Texas may look normal in southern California. In some cultures, psychological distress is more likely to be experienced as physical symptoms, while in others it is expressed as emotion. Patients with limited English-speaking skills may have trouble communicating with clinicians who do not understand their native language. Or the culture of the clinician may cause him or her to misinterpret signs and symptoms in someone from a different culture.

Accuracy can be a very real problem in diagnosing bipolar disorder. However, if you've been diagnosed by several different clinicians as having bipolar disorder and you have experienced the symptoms described in Chapters 1 through 4, there is a good chance that your diagnosis is accurate. If, despite a lot of evidence, you are still fighting the diagnosis, maybe it's time to reexamine the facts and take charge of your mood swings.

Receiving a Diagnosis

It is one thing to understand what a doctor means when he or she says that you have bipolar disorder. It's another to find it acceptable and believable. Agreeing with a diagnosis of bipolar disorder means accepting not only that you have a mental illness, but also that you have one that will require lifelong treatment. This is a lot to swallow at one time. It is natural to resist the idea, say that the doctor is wrong, explain away the symptoms as due to stress or too much partying, or believe that you're just going through a phase.

If you do not want to be given a diagnosis of bipolar disorder, you might not be completely honest with the doctor about your symptoms. You might downplay mood swings and changes in your behavior that occurred when manic or depressed. In this case, your lack of acceptance can interfere with the diagnostic process. And if you know that you have been less than completely forthright in the information you have given and the diagnosis still comes out to be bipolar disorder, you will question the accuracy of the diagnosis.

Doesn't Everyone Have Mood Swings?

Mood swings vary greatly in severity, as the figure below shows. On the low end of severity is the normal range of human experience, where people feel down when bad things happen and feel elated when good things happen. These states are usually temporary and relate specifically to an event. When the event is over, the mood returns to normal or neutral. There are also some people who are moody by nature. They do not have the physical symptoms of depression or mania; they are just cranky or temperamental. They do not have a mental illness, but they are different from the happy go-lucky type. Then there are those who are perky, optimistic, and hopeful, even in the face of adversity. They are not manic, just good-natured.

Moving up the scale in severity are people whose mood is worsened by physical problems or stress. The best example is premenstrual syndrome, or PMS. Women who have PMS have a definite drop in their mood that can last a week or so prior to starting their periods and can linger for a few days afterward. It is caused by changes in hormone levels, bloating, pain, and other physical discomforts, but it goes away as predictably as it arrives. Low blood sugar can also cause moodiness for anyone but is more severe in those who have diabetes. Seasonal allergy attacks can cause irritability until symptoms subside, as can other physical

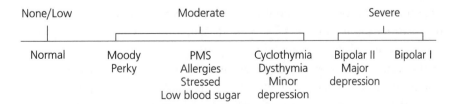

Range of severity of mood swings.

discomforts such as rashes or pain. Stress alters mood, causing irritability, anxiety, sadness, and frustration. If the stressful problem persists, the negative mood state persists. Stress can cause some of the symptoms of bipolar disorder, such as irritability and insomnia, in people who do not have the illness.

More severe are the diagnosable mood disorders. *Diagnosable* means that they meet criteria set out in DSM-5. Dysthymia or dysthymic disorder is a chronic but usually mild depression that can be lifelong. It is more than being moody, but not as severe as major depression. In dysthymia, people have a low mood at least half the time and a few of the physical features of major depression or low self-esteem. People who have dysthymia can also have periods of major depression during the course of their life. When their major depression is over, they usually go back to being dysthymic.

Cyclothymia is a mild form of bipolar disorder and is also lifelong. Ups that look like hypomania and downs that are fairly mild alternate throughout a person's life. What looks like cyclothymia could also be the beginnings of the development of bipolar disorder.

Minor depression is also called *unspecified depressive disorder* and is diagnosed when a person has a sad mood and a few of the physical symptoms listed under major depression but falls short of the five symptoms needed to diagnose major depression. Minor depression is often triggered by a stressful event, lasts for a short while until the person gets over the event, and usually remits without treatment.

Bipolar II and major depression vary greatly in severity, and although they are listed on the continuum as less severe than bipolar I disorder, they can be just as chronic and cause just as much misery. Major depression has already been described. Once it occurs, it tends to recur, sometimes related to distressing events and sometimes for no reason at all. It can also be chronic, lasting years at a time with no relief.

Bipolar II disorder is defined as having periods of major depression and periods of hypomania. Hypomania is a less severe state of mania (*hypo-* means "less than" or "under"). Hypomanic episodes cause most of the symptoms already described. However, when in this state, most people are still fully aware of the changes they are going through, and they don't act on the urges or impulses that are going through their minds. What best distinguishes mania from hypomania is the amount of impairment it causes. Mania is usually diagnosed when the symptoms are present and are severe enough to cause significant problems or are severe enough that you might need to be hospitalized to stay safe. These problems can include going into significant debt due to spending sprees, sexual promiscuity that causes relationship problems or health problems, reckless driving that causes accidents, impulsively quitting a job without a plan to support yourself, or even running away from home and neglecting your responsibilities. In contrast, during a hypomanic episode, you may have the symptoms listed for mania and also the desire to run away, spend money, or have an affair, but you stay in control and don't take those actions.

Now that you have read about the many different types of mood swings, you may be able to better understand why your doctor and therapists think you have bipolar disorder instead of just run-of-the-mill mood changes. If you think your symptoms would be better explained as a different disorder, talk it over with your doctor or therapist.

What's Next?

The goal of this chapter was to help you understand how clinicians view the symptoms of depression, mania, and hypomania and the challenges that they face in making a correct diagnosis. Your personal experience with symptoms may be very different from the descriptions in this chapter. Chapter 3 will help you identify your personal pattern of symptoms and how they differ from the real you. Take time to complete the exercises in Chapter 3. They set the stage for the exercises in the remaining chapters.

3

Distinguish Symptoms
from the Real You

In this chapter you will:

✓ Learn about the subtle signs of depression and mania.

✓ Figure out how your moods and symptoms change over time.

✓ Distinguish between a symptom and the real you.

As you know, the mood swings and other symptoms of bipolar disorder can come and go throughout your life. There are, however, things you can do to manage severe symptoms and even stop them from recurring. To do this, you need to know when symptoms are beginning to emerge. Having an early warning system, like the kind used to track storms, can alert you to use the strategies in this workbook along with medications to stop the symptoms before they become severe. Whether you have bipolar I disorder or less severe forms of mood swings, you can benefit from creating an early warning system even if your highs and lows are few and far between.

The exercises in this chapter will help you become more aware of changes in your mood, thoughts, and actions so that you have a chance to intervene. For example, long before you're in a full episode of mania, you might become irritable and tense, each day having less and less patience with people. Noises might bother you more and more. And your sleep could slowly worsen from mild insomnia to total sleeplessness. Depression can also come on slowly. You may initially experience a drop in your energy level or difficulty motivating yourself at work, home, or school. Your interest in being around other people may lessen until you find yourself isolated from friends and family members. Learning how your symptoms progress will prepare you to intervene when the symptoms return.

How Symptoms of Depression and Mania Progress

The symptoms of depression and mania are obvious and easy to recognize when severe. But usually there are subtle signs that your mood is changing long before it becomes noticeable to others. The goal is to learn to recognize subtle changes as early as possible. The quicker you notice them, the quicker you can take action to stop them.

The table in Exercise 3.1 lists common symptoms of depression along with examples of how they might appear in their mild or moderate forms (see p. 32). When episodes of depression start, you might, for example, feel only a little low or blue, but as the episode worsens, your low feeling might cause you to cry more easily than usual. In severe depression, the low mood will often worsen into severe sadness. Use Exercise 3.1 to make note of the symptoms of depression you have experienced. You may download and print additional copies of this worksheet from *www.guilford.com/basco2-forms* and add them to your workbook as needed.

The table in Exercise 3.2 lists common symptoms of mania in their mild, moderate, and severe forms (see p. 33). For example, you might be able to recognize irritability as a severe symptom, but this shift in mood usually starts with a milder symptom such as impatience or anxiety. As it progresses, your irritation might begin to show as you become more easily angered than usual. Read through this table. If you have only had hypomania and never mania, you have probably only experienced these symptoms in their mild or moderate forms. Use Exercise 3.2 to make note of the symptoms of mania or hypomania that you have experienced. You may download and print additional copies of this worksheet from *www.guilford. com/basco2-forms* and add them to your workbook as needed.

Although symptoms do not always take the same shape when they recur, it is possible that you will have similar symptoms in the future. In mania, you can experience euphoria and the other symptoms that go along with a positive mood or you can have an irritable mania where the symptoms may be more negative.

The Mood Symptoms Worksheet

Most people who have been through multiple episodes of depression and mania have difficulty distinguishing symptoms of depression from symptoms of mania. This is because there are some symptoms that are common to both states, such as having trouble sleeping or being irritable. Also when people are having a recurrence of symptoms they just feel bad in general and are fearful of what lies ahead of them. The reason it is important to know the difference between the onset of mania and the onset of depression is that the treatments you will apply to stop the symptoms from worsening are going to be different.

Your Common Symptoms of Depression

As you read through the list of common symptoms of depression, circle the ones that you have experienced in the past.

Mild form of symptom	Moderate form of symptom	Severe symptom of depression
Blue, down, or neutral mood	*Cry more easily*	**Severe sadness**
Not in the mood to socialize	*Less involved with others*	**Lack of interest in usual activities**
Usual activities are not as much fun as expected	*Have fun until activity is over*	**Decreased pleasure**
Blame self more readily when things go wrong; see own faults	*Self-critical*	**Excessive and inappropriate guilt**
Not as hungry as usual; can skip meals occasionally and not feel hungry	*Eating brings less pleasure*	**Decreased appetite**
Clothes fit slightly looser, no big weight loss (e.g., 1–3 pounds)	*Noticeable weight loss*	**Significant weight loss**
Sleep seems less restful; ruminating at bedtime; falling asleep takes a little longer	*Takes much longer to fall asleep; wake up briefly during the night*	**Insomnia—cannot fall asleep easily, wake up during the night and stay awake**
Lose interest in tasks such as reading; get frustrated with tasks that are lengthy	*Must reread text; thoughts cannot be focused well*	**Impaired concentration**
Feel as if you are moving slowly; not mentally sharp	*Slowness in movement is noticeable to others; long pauses before answering questions*	**Psychomotor retardation**
Wish pain would go away; thoughts of running away; pessimistic	*Thoughts that life may not be worth living; hopeless; can't imagine feeling better*	**Suicidal ideas or attempts; not caring if you died**
Self-doubt; some self-criticism	*Low self-esteem, dislike appearance, feel like a loser*	**Feelings of worthlessness**

As you read through the list of common symptoms of mania, circle the ones that you have experienced.

Mild form of symptom	Moderate form of symptom	Severe symptom of mania
Everything seems like a hassle; impatience or anxiety	More easily angered	Irritability
Happier than usual, positive outlook	Increased laughter and joking	Euphoric mood; on top of the world
More talkative, better sense of humor	In the mood to socialize and talk with others	Pressured or rapid speech
More thoughts; mentally sharp, quick; lose focus	Disorganized thinking, poor concentration	Racing thoughts
More self-confident than usual, less pessimistic	Feeling smart, not afraid to try, overly optimistic	Grandiosity—delusions of grandeur
Creative ideas, new interests; change sounds good.	Plan to make changes; disorganized in actions, drinking or smoking more	Disorganized activity; starting more things than finishing
Fidgety; nervous behaviors like nail biting	Restless, preferring movement over sedentary activities	Psychomotor agitation; cannot sit still
Not as effective at work, having trouble keeping mind on tasks	Not completing tasks, late for work, annoying others	Cannot complete usual work or home activities
Uncomfortable with other people	Suspicious	Paranoia
More sexually interested	Sexual dreams, seeking out or noticing sexual stimulation	Increased sex drive, seek out sexual activity, more promiscuous
Notice sounds and annoying people, lose train of thought	Noises seem louder, colors seem brighter, mind wanders easily; need quieter environment to focus thoughts	Distractibility—have to work hard to focus thoughts or cannot focus thoughts at all

The goal of the Mood Symptoms Worksheet is to help you begin to distinguish between symptoms of depression and symptoms of mania. The Mood Symptoms Worksheet on the facing page has three columns to fill in. One is for describing what you are like when manic, the second is for symptoms of depression, and the third column is for describing what you are like when you are not having symptoms. Think about each category of symptom and describe how it differs when you are depressed, when you are manic, and when you are feeling OK. For example, what is your mood like when you are depressed? Are you sad or blue? How is it different when you are manic? Do you get happy or irritable? What is your usual mood when you are not having a lot of symptoms? Are you usually in a pretty good mood? Are you cranky by nature? Do you feel bored most of the time?

Even for symptoms like insomnia that happen during depression and mania, you can probably tell the difference between these two types of sleeplessness. In depression you may have trouble falling asleep even though you are exhausted. When you wake up in the morning, you are still tired. In mania, you may have too much energy to settle down to fall asleep, and when you wake up in the morning you may feel rested and ready to go.

Try to fill in the Mood Symptoms Worksheet in Exercise 3.3 with your own examples. You can refer back to the items you circled in the lists of manic and depressive symptoms in the previous section. Try to resist writing in "good" or "bad" for each category on the sheet. Instead, try to describe the symptom. For example, under "mood," describe the type of mood you have when you are feeling depressed (e.g., blue, sad, hopeless, angry, anxious, bored, or miserable). Under the category of sleep habits, write in how many hours of sleep you get or what kind of trouble you have with your sleep (e.g., can't fall asleep, wake up multiple times, wake up too early and can't go back to sleep).

When you have finished your worksheet, ask your family members or friends to share their observations of the ways they think you change when you are becoming depressed or manic. Add these additional symptoms to the list. You may not be able to fill in each box today, but as you learn more about yourself, go back and fill in the symptoms you have begun to notice. You may download and print additional copies of this worksheet from *www.guilford.com/basco2-forms* and add them to your workbook as needed.

Paul completed the Mood Symptoms Worksheet, part of which is shown on page 37. He had not previously thought about how he changed from feeling fine to feeling up or depressed. Seeing his own words on the worksheet helped him think about his mood swings differently. Mood swings are not just about his mood. He changes in a number of ways. Some of the changes are more noticeable to him than others, such as his sleep patterns. He can use these more noticeable changes as cues that he is switching into a low of depression or a high of mania.

Ways to Use Your Mood Symptoms Worksheet

Suggestion 1

The symptoms you have listed are your warning signs that depression or mania may be returning. These are the symptoms to watch for on a regular basis. If you notice any of the

Mood Symptoms Worksheet

Category	When manic or hypomanic	When depressed or down	When feeling OK, or like my usual self
Mood			
Attitude toward self			
Self-confidence			
Usual activities			
Social activity			
Sleep habits			
Appetite/eating habits			
Concentration			
Speed of thought			
Creativity			
Interest in having fun			

(cont.)

From *The Bipolar Workbook, Second Edition*. Copyright 2015 by The Guilford Press.

Category	When manic or hypomanic	When depressed or down	When feeling OK, or like my usual self
Restlessness			
Sense of humor			
Energy level			
How noise affects you			
Outlook on the future			
Speech patterns			
Decision-making ability			
Concern for others			
Thoughts about death			
Ability to function			
Other areas:			

	PAUL'S EXAMPLE Mood Symptoms Worksheet		
Category	**When manic or hypomanic**	**When depressed or down**	**When feeling OK, or like my usual self**
Mood	Irritable.	Sad.	Content.
Attitude toward self	I'm the only one with a brain.	I hate myself.	I'm OK.
Self-confidence	Very self-confident.	No confidence.	I think I am capable of a lot.
Usual activities	Starting but not finishing tasks.	Lie in bed or watch TV.	Work. Clean house. Exercise.
Social activity	Can't stand to be around people.	I don't want anyone to see me.	Visit with friends and family.
Sleep habits	4 hours each night.	Sleep all the time.	7–8 hours of sleep.
Appetite/eating habits	I forget to eat.	I'm not hungry.	I like to eat.
Concentration	Can't hold on to thoughts.	Stare at a page, but can't read.	Pretty good. I can read the paper.
Speed of thought	Fast and disorganized	My mind is slow and sluggish.	I'm usually a quick thinker.
Creativity	Very creative until I reach my peak.	No creative thoughts.	Can be creative at home.
Interest in having fun	I'm more likely to go out.	Not interested.	I like having fun with my friends.
Restlessness	Very hard to sit still.	I don't want to move off couch.	I like to be busy and keep moving.
Sense of humor	More sarcastic.	Nothing is funny.	Like to tell jokes.
Energy level	High. Nervous energy.	None.	Enough to get things done.
How noise affects you	Noises get on my nerves.	I don't hear what's going on around me.	It doesn't usually bother me.

warning signs, call your doctor for help and take the precautions you have learned for keeping your symptoms under control.

Suggestion 2

Give a copy of your Mood Symptoms Worksheet to your doctor and therapist. That will help them understand you better and will help them recognize changes in you that you might not notice.

Suggestion 3

Give a copy of the worksheet to family members who live with you and can help you monitor your symptoms.

Suggestion 4

If you think you may be having a return of symptoms but are not certain, read through the list to see how many symptoms you are having. If you have a few symptoms that are mild, do what you can to keep them from worsening.

Suggestion 5

Here are some questions to ask yourself. If the answer to any is "yes," take action to fix the problem and keep the symptom from worsening.

- "Have I been taking my medication regularly and at the right dose?"
- "Have I been getting enough sleep at night? What adjustments do I need to make?"
- "Am I doing anything that could make matters worse?"
- "Are my symptoms getting worse each day?"
- "Do I need some help? Who should I call?"
- "Is there something I could do today to help myself feel better? Could I change my negative thinking, slow down, get some rest, or take positive actions toward solving a problem?"
- "Should I start monitoring my mood daily?"

Lost Track of the Real You?

If you have struggled with mood swings for a long time, you may find it hard to fill in the column of Exercise 3.3 that is labeled "When feeling OK, or like my usual self." The things that are part of your personality and not a symptom of a mood swing tend to be fairly consistent over time. For example, your values, preferences, tastes, faith, feelings about loved ones, job skills, intelligence, and philosophy of life are all part of the real you.

Symptoms of bipolar disorder and other types of mood swings can mask the real you. For example, Amanda is a problem solver at work. When she is depressed, however, she gets overwhelmed by the smallest problems and forgets that she is quite capable of analyzing situations, figuring out what needs to be done, and taking action. Her symptoms muddle her thinking and keep her from using her excellent problem-solving skills.

Some personality traits can make you more vulnerable when mood swings occur. Maria is a very kind person and is sensitive to the needs of others. In her family, Maria is the one who remembers to send birthday cards, takes flowers to her grandmother when she is not feeling well, and takes in stray kittens. It makes Maria feel good to do these things, and she appreciates it when others do kind things for her. She is aware that other people in her family do not share this trait, and she tries not to feel offended when they forget her birthday or fail to compliment her on a new hairstyle or outfit.

When Maria is manic, her kindness makes her vulnerable to excessive spending. She gets the urge to shop, sees things that she thinks others would like, and buys them. Her friends who know about her bipolar disorder recognize the excessive gift purchases as a symptom, but Maria doesn't see it until the credit card bill comes in the mail.

When Maria is depressed, her thoughtfulness makes her vulnerable when people do not make time to do kind things for her. She is not likely to get a card or even a phone call from her family even if she has made it clear that she is not feeling well. On the contrary, it seems to Maria that during these times they continue to make demands on her time: "Can you pick up a cake for your sister's baby shower? You know where to get the best cakes." "Let Maria wrap the gift. She can make it look so pretty." "Maria, pick up your grandmother and bring her to the house for dinner. You can fit her wheelchair in your truck." What Maria hears is that no one cares that she is depressed.

Conversely, your personality characteristics can also help you cope during severe mood swings. Joe has a very strong work ethic. He takes pride in his work and believes that it is important to fulfill his commitments on the job even if he is not feeling his best. When Joe feels pulled into another period of depression, his determination at work helps him power through the bad days. He stays busy as a way of ignoring his sad feelings and negative thoughts. He does simple tasks if he can't concentrate, and he makes an effort to interact with positive people. His drive to work hard is greater than the seductive feeling of lethargy that makes him want to retreat to his chair and watch TV all day.

Paul's strength is in his determination to not let his bipolar disorder control his life. He knows he has an illness, and he understands that he has to take medication to control it. He also believes that there is more to him than just an illness. He will not let his diagnosis define him. These strengths help him cope when his symptoms begin to emerge. He is not afraid to ask for help from his doctor or his family. He makes sure that he takes his medication every day. He grew up with a friend who has diabetes and needs insulin injections every day. Paul sees his illness in the same way—taking medications every day keeps him healthy.

As you work to gain control over your mood swings, it is important not only to recognize your symptoms but also to be aware of your strengths and weaknesses. Knowing your strengths is a tool. You can use them to get through difficult days when medications alone do not make you feel better. Awareness of your weaknesses can help you avoid trouble if you learn to recognize how they may be contributing to your mood swings.

What Are Your Strengths?

During bouts of depression it may be hard for you to answer this question. Your negative mood will make you aware of your weaknesses, everything you don't like about yourself, and your regrets or failures. During periods of irritable mania or hypomania, you may have the same problem.

Your strengths include positive character traits. For Maria a strength is her kindness, and for Joe it is his strong work ethic. A strength can also be an ability such as intelligence or a good sense of humor. One of Amanda's strengths is that she is decisive even in tough situations. That makes her a good nurse. Miguel loves to work on cars. His strengths include the patience and eye for detail needed to take apart and put together car engines. Raquel's strength is her self-awareness. She knows when her symptoms are influencing her actions.

What are your strengths? How might they help you cope when mood swings occur? Use Exercise 3.4 to remind yourself of your strengths. A few categories have been included to get you started. If one of your strengths is that you are comfortable talking to people, ask others to help you with this exercise. If your strength is that you take time to think things through before making a decision, come back to this exercise after you have had some time to think about it. If you are depressed and do not see any of your strengths, come back to this exercise when you are feeling better or get your therapist or other mental health provider to help you.

After you have completed your inventory of personal strengths, take some time to think about how they help you cope with your mood swings. Maria, for example, draws strength from her faith in God and from the people in her life. When she is feeling down, she prays for support. She also talks to her friends about it. It helps Maria to know that her family loves her, but she doesn't tell them about her depression because they would worry too much about her. She can take care of herself, another one of her strengths. Instead of calling her mother, she calls her counselor or makes an appointment with her psychiatrist.

Throughout this workbook you will learn many new ways to cope with mood swings. As you gain these new skills you can add them to your list of personal strengths. A list of strengths can remind you that you have many abilities that can be used to make it through difficult times.

Take time to create a to-do list with Exercise 3.5 on page 43 and use it as a reminder when you need help to cope with your highs and lows.

Inventory of Personal Strengths

Next to each category of strengths, make a note about your personal strengths. Include strengths that you have had in the past but may not be using at present.

Type of strength	Your examples
Mental abilities (e.g., good memory, common sense)	
Physical abilities (e.g., sleep well, high energy)	
Personality characteristics (e.g., don't give up easily)	
People skills (e.g., patience, good listener)	
Work skills (e.g., computer skills, get along with others at work)	
Healthy habits (e.g., don't eat sweets, stopped smoking)	
Knowledge (e.g., read about medications, know where to go for help)	
Talents (e.g., can make people laugh)	
Experience (e.g., been through difficult times, know now to survive)	
Other strengths	

Inventory of Personal Strengths

Type of strength	Your examples
Mental abilities (e.g., good memory, common sense)	I have a very good memory. I think I have good common sense.
Physical abilities (e.g., sleep well, high energy)	I can't think of any. I'm not in shape right now.
Personality characteristics (e.g., don't give up easily)	I'm a nice person. I care about others. I am trustworthy.
People skills (e.g., patience, good listener)	I treat people the way I would want to be treated. I call people or send cards for their birthdays. I show concern for others even if they do not show concern for me.
Work skills (e.g., computer skills, get along with others at work)	I'm the detail person at work. I catch mistakes and fix them. People come to me to check their work.
Healthy habits (e.g., don't eat sweets, stopped smoking)	I don't smoke, but I eat too many sweets. Sometimes I exercise, but not regularly.
Knowledge (e.g., read about medications, know where to go for help)	I read about my illness. I look up my medications on the Internet.
Talents (e.g., can make people laugh)	I'm very creative. I make things that amaze people like picture frames and Christmas ornaments.
Experience (e.g., been through difficult times, know now to survive)	I know when I am depressed. I know how to keep it to myself and not bother others with it.
Other strengths	I have faith in God.
	I have a good family that loves me.
	I have good friends that care about me.
	I'm not stupid. I know what I need to do to take care of myself.
	I'm independent. I can take care of myself.

A To-Do List for Symptom Control

Select from the strengths you listed in Exercise 3.4 those that have been most helpful in managing your highs and lows. Create a to-do list that reminds you when to use your strengths and how they can help.

Strengths that help me cope	When it might be helpful	How it can help

MARIA'S EXAMPLE **A To-Do List for Symptom Control**

Strengths that help me cope	When it might be helpful	How it can help
The people who support me	*When my head is full of negative thoughts*	*They remind me that I am not stupid, ugly, or hopeless even if I feel that way.*
My faith in God	*When I am thinking of death*	*Keeps me from seriously considering suicide*
My common sense	*When I think about doing stupid things like spending too much money on useless things*	*My common sense tells me that wanting to spend money is a symptom of hypomania and not a real need.*

What's Next?

The goal of this chapter was to help you recognize symptoms of depression and mania and begin to understand how they differ from the real you. The exercises provided you with an opportunity for self-reflection and a chance to get input from others on what you are like when you have symptoms of bipolar disorder. Your work on the exercises in this chapter will prepare you for the next chapter, where you will learn to monitor your symptoms over time so that you can catch mood swings before they become severe.

Step 2

See It Coming

4

Recognize and Label
Your Moods

In this chapter you will:

✓ Find out why it is important to monitor your mood swings.

✓ Begin to recognize and label your mood.

✓ Learn how to track your mood swings.

Not everyone can recognize his or her own mood swings, at least not right away. It can be much easier to recognize changes in other people's moods than in your own mood. You can see it in their facial expressions or body language. You can hear it in their tone of voice, choice of words, how loudly they speak, or when they shut down and say nothing at all. You can even judge their mood by their actions. It is harder, however, to notice the same changes in yourself.

You can learn to listen for the changes in your tone and choice of words that signal a shift in your mood. Joe, for example, tells dirty jokes at work when he is getting manic. He is a supervisor and knows it's inappropriate, but he doesn't realize he's doing it until he notices the looks on the faces of those around him. Raquel says that her therapist knows she is getting manic by the way she walks across the waiting room. The extra bounce in her step and the bigger-than-usual smile on her face give her away every time.

You can learn to identify sensations in your body that are clues to your mood. For example, you can catch yourself staring at the ground when you walk or feel a frown on your face when you are low. You might notice a headache from tensing your face or furrowing your brow when you're worried. Your actions can also give you clues—hitting the snooze button too many times or turning off the alarm clock and staying in bed when you're not in the mood to face the day.

As described in Chapter 3, the key to controlling your mood symptoms is recognizing when it is time to intervene. This requires the development of greater self-awareness. The goal of this chapter is to help you become more aware of subtle changes in your feelings and actions that signal a recurrence of depression or mania. In Chapter 3 you read about mild, moderate, and severe symptoms of depression and mania. In this chapter, the focus is on subtler signs.

If you are already aware of the subtle signs of a mood swing and are sensitive to those changes, you may want to skim the first part of this chapter and focus more attention on the Mood Graphs toward the end. The exercises in this chapter were designed for people who do not always realize they are becoming depressed, hypomanic, or manic. First you will learn simple concepts such as labeling your mood and then advance to daily symptom monitoring.

First You Have to Know Yourself

Some people know themselves well. They are aware of the subtle changes in their moods. They can describe many different types of good moods and bad moods. Not everyone, however, has this level of self-awareness. How about you? When people ask you how you feel, do you tend to just say either good or bad? If so, you may need to do the next exercise.

In Exercise 4.1 below, try to describe how it feels when you are in a good mood and in a bad mood. If it has been a while since you have experienced either one, try to recall the last time your mood swung in either direction.

EXERCISE 4.1 Owning My Mood	
In the spaces below, try to describe what it feels like to be in a good and bad mood.	
When I am in a good mood, I would describe it as:	**Some examples include:**
	joyful, happy, excited, calm, peaceful, content, neutral, relieved, worry-free, playful, silly, fun
When I am in a bad mood, I would describe it as:	**Some examples include:**
	sad, blue, down, regretful, tearful, upset, angry, irritable, annoyed, worried, stressed, fearful

If you have trouble with Exercise 4.1, ask others to help you. Let them tell you about the last time they saw you in what seemed to be a good mood. How would they have described you? Do the same for bad moods. If you don't have anyone you can ask, try the exercise on someone you know or a character you have seen on a television show. How would you describe their good moods and bad moods? Pay attention to the signs that tell you about their mood. Maybe you can learn to recognize these signs in yourself.

Most people experience changes in their moods from day to day or even from hour to hour, depending on the circumstances. Owning your mood means recognizing those fluctuations in mood, being able to label them, and learning how to manage them. Some people are more skilled than others in recognizing changes in their mood. Exercise 4.2 below will test your self-awareness.

Raquel is usually aware of when her mood is dropping, but she does not have the same kind of awareness when her mood is going up—when she is getting hypomanic or manic. She filled out Exercise 4.2 when she was hypomanic. You can see on the next page that she recognized her mood was somewhere between neutral and good, but her description does not sound like hypomania. She understands what it means to feel bad or sad, but she thinks that feeling high is normal for her. When her mood is neutral—not up or down—she thinks this is depression. She has lost her ability to see the difference.

Because depression feels so awful and hypomania and mania can feel good, people get confused about what it means to be normal. Some may mistake hypomanic feelings for

---

EXERCISE 4.2   How Would You Describe Your Mood Today?

Step 1: Mark a spot on the line that best describes your mood today.

_____

Bad   Neutral/Not Bad or Good   Good

Step 2: Try to put a label on your mood. Do any of the words in Exercise 4.1 apply?
Today my mood is best described as:

Step 3: How can you tell? What do your thoughts, sensations, or actions tell you about your mood?
I know my mood is _____ because:

RAQUEL'S EXAMPLE   How Would You Describe Your Mood Today?

Step 1: Mark a spot on the line that best describes your mood today.

—————————————————————✕————————————————————

Bad   Neutral/Not Bad or Good   Good

Step 2: Try to put a label on your mood. Do any of the words in Exercise 4.1 apply?
Today my mood is best described as:

outstanding, better than neutral, but not high

Step 3: How can you tell? What do your thoughts, sensations, or actions tell you about your mood?
I know my mood is _____*outstanding*_____ because:

I'm not mad at anyone today. I'm not stressed out. I'm feeling really good. I'm getting a lot done.

normal feelings because in that state they don't feel bad. This is Raquel's problem. She misses the warning signs of mania because she thinks that she is just feeling "normal."

She is not alone. A lot of people make this mistake. In fact, some people associate feeling neutral—not up or down—with being depressed. The absence of intense feelings seems foreign to them; they don't like it. They don't realize that people who do not have bipolar disorder feel neutral a lot of the time.

Gaining Self-Awareness

For many people, their moods are tied to their surroundings and the people around them. People can leave you feeling good or bad. Places can have the same effect. Paul gets irritated every time he has to go to the post office. The lines are long, and it seems to him that the people who work at his post office don't care about providing good service. His mood becomes irritable at the thought of having to pick up or drop off a package. Even when he starts off the day in a good mood, he is annoyed by the time he leaves the house to head to the post office.

Paul's girlfriend, Angie, does not think it has much to do with the post office. She notices that when Paul's mood is a little low, going to places where he has to stand in line even for a short while seems overwhelming to him. He blames it on the people there, but Angie can see that the bad mood starts with him.

Joe's wife, Sarah, is similar in this regard. She hates visiting with Joe's stepmother. She thinks the woman hates her. Just thinking about having to visit puts Sarah in a bad mood. From Joe's point of view, Sarah's mood is tied to the chronic pain in her back. Joe's stepmother hasn't always been tactful about this. In the past, she made comments suggesting that Sarah's pain was all in her head. Joe corrected his stepmother and convinced her to keep her opinions to herself, but Sarah won't let it go. She doesn't see that anticipating a visit with Joe's stepmother puts her in a bad mood because she is feeling uncomfortable and she will not let go of the past.

Moods and experiences are closely tied to one another. If you are in a bad mood, you can have negative interactions with others. Likewise, bad situations can ruin a perfectly good mood. Often, it is hard to tell which came first.

It is human nature to try to make sense of unpleasant events by assigning blame to the person or thing you think caused it to happen. If you have limited self-awareness of the ways in which bipolar disorder affects you, it is easy to draw the wrong conclusion and attribute bad feelings to other people or events rather than to your mood swings. There are ways that you can learn to become more self-aware.

Mood Signs

Except for when you are depressed, it's pretty normal to spend your time moving from activity to activity without really stopping to think about how you feel. It starts when you get up in the morning and start your day. When you are depressed, you are keenly aware as soon as you wake up that you are feeling lousy and that it is going to be a bad day. The feeling is hard to miss. Other emotions, however, are more subtle or difficult to detect.

People who are manic are often not aware of it. When you're irritable or angry, you think it is someone else's fault. Worry or anxiety is generally tied to a problem you are facing or an event that scares you. These are examples of times when you might not be aware of your mood because you attribute it to something outside of you—it is someone or something else's fault. Exercise 4.3 on page 52 poses some questions about your feelings and mood. Take a moment and think about each one. Maybe you are more aware of your feelings than you think. You just need to pay closer attention and gather a few clues to begin to recognize subtle changes that signal the next mood swing. After each question there is an example of how others might answer the question.

If you answered yes to any of the questions in Exercise 4.3, perhaps you could use some help to recognize your mood swings. It begins with paying attention, making mental notes about how you feel, and learning to connect your experiences with your mood. Exercise 4.4 on page 54 can help you get started.

EXERCISE 4.3 Finding Clues to Your Mood

1. Can you tell by your actions how you are really feeling?

   Joe knows he is in a bad mood when he finds himself dropping things or forgetting things at work. He makes mistakes and gets mad at himself. That's how he knows that he is irritable. **How about you?**

2. Have there been times when you are not aware of your mood until you hear yourself react to another person?

   Paul doesn't realize that he is feeling anxious until he hears his girlfriend repeatedly say, "It'll be all right. There's nothing to worry about." He feels himself getting mad at her when the problem is really that he is stressing out over something small. **Do you do that?**

3. Do other people claim to know your mood by the look on your face even when you think you are fine?

   Tommy's mom claims she knows her son better than he knows himself. When she says this, he feels annoyed. Later, he realizes that she is right. She can tell by his body language when he is feeling down. He hates it when she's right. **Do you know someone like that?**

4. Is it hard for you to tell that you are depressed until you have trouble functioning?

   Amanda doesn't see that she is slipping into depression until she realizes how behind she is at home. She gets mad at her husband for not helping and at the kids for making a mess. It takes her a while to realize that her house is a mess because she has been spending more time than usual in front of the television or in bed. **Does that sound like you?**

Monitoring Your Mood

There are several reasons to monitor your mood or other symptoms regularly. For example, becoming more tuned in to your daily changes in mood will help you identify any specific factors that consistently affect your mood. For example, do you seem to get depressed on rainy days or at the times when you have nothing to do? Do you start to get hyper or manic when there is too much noise or confusion or when you haven't had enough sleep?

You can keep track of mania, hypomania, or depression by monitoring your mood regularly or by watching for other signs or symptoms that mark the beginning of an episode.

Some people notice changes in their sleep habits first; some find it difficult to concentrate; others find themselves getting more easily annoyed with others.

When he's getting depressed, Paul sleeps when he is not at work. Amanda starts worrying a lot more. Raquel is sentimental and cries when watching TV commercials. When he's getting manic, Tommy is not certain what happens, because he has had bipolar disorder for only a short time, but his friends have told him that he wants to party all night. His mom says that he picks fights with her. Amanda knows she's getting manic when her house is spotlessly clean.

Mood Graphs

In Exercise 4.4 on the next page you will find a Mood Graph. It is designed so that you can rate your mood each day for 1 week. The scale in the first column goes from +5 at the top, representing severe mania, to –5 at the bottom, representing severe depression. A rating of 0 in the middle represents a neutral mood, not good or bad.

Circle a dot each day next to the rating that best describes your mood. At the end of the week, connect the dots to see how your mood has fluctuated. At the bottom of the graph, make notes about any circumstances that might be associated with a change in your mood. Perhaps you forgot to take your medications for a few days, were unable to sleep, or were under a great deal of stress. These clues will help you better understand what causes your mood to change and your symptoms to return.

You may download and print additional copies of the Mood Graph from *www.guilford. com/basco2-forms* and add them to your workbook as needed.

Symptom Tracking

What changes do you notice first when you are getting depressed? What changes do you notice first when you are getting manic? Look over your Mood Symptoms Worksheet on pages 35 and 36 and pick out the category of symptom that you are likely to notice first.

For some people, it's easier to monitor physical symptoms, sleep habits, or changes in thinking than to monitor their mood. Pick a symptom that you would notice changing if you were beginning an episode of depression or mania and write it in on the Symptom Graph on page 56 (Exercise 4.5). Here are some common examples:

Monitor changes in *energy level*: +5 means tremendous energy, cannot sit still
  0 means normal levels of energy
  –5 means no energy at all, cannot move

Monitor changes in *concentration*: +5 means so many thoughts you can't speak
  0 means normal levels of concentration
  –5 means thinking is extremely slow

Use this worksheet to track your mood each day.								
Week of:	**Plan**	**Sun**	**Mon**	**Tues**	**Wed**	**Thur**	**Fri**	**Sat**
Manic **+5** Not sleeping, psychotic	*Go to the hospital*	●	●	●	●	●	●	●
+4 Manic, poor judgment		●	●	●	●	●	●	●
+3 Hypomanic	*Call the doctor*	●	●	●	●	●	●	●
+2 Energized	*Take action*	●	●	●	●	●	●	●
+1 Hyper, happy	*Watch closely*	●	●	●	●	●	●	●
0 Normal		●	●	●	●	●	●	●
−1 Low, down	*Watch closely*	●	●	●	●	●	●	●
−2 Sad	*Take action*	●	●	●	●	●	●	●
−3 Depressed	*Call the doctor*	●	●	●	●	●	●	●
−4 Immobilized		●	●	●	●	●	●	●
−5 Suicidal **Depressed**	*Go to the hospital*	●	●	●	●	●	●	●

What caused the mood shift?

Monitor changes in *self-esteem*:   +5 means *"I think I'm a god"*
                                                    0 means self-esteem is OK
                                                    –5 means *"I hate myself," "I have no value"*

After you've picked a category, write in a word that would describe what the category would look like at each level, from –5 to +5. For example, if you were measuring energy level changes, you might write "tired" next to –2 and "hyper" next to +2. Monitor changes each day and mark them on the graph.

Circle a dot each day next to the rating that best describes the intensity of the symptom you are tracking. At the end of the week, connect the dots to see how your symptoms have fluctuated. At the bottom of the graph, make notes about any circumstances that might be associated with a change in your symptom. Perhaps you forgot to take your medications for a few days, were unable to sleep, or were under a great deal of stress. These clues will help you better understand what causes your mood to change and your symptoms to return.

You may download and print extra copies of the Symptom Graph from *www.guilford. com/basco2-forms* and add them to your workbook as needed.

Ways to Use Your Mood and Symptom Graphs

- The primary goal of the Mood Graph is to identify recurrence of symptoms when they are beginning. This can be accomplished by being mindful of mild mood shifts. If you make a habit of rating your mood each day, you will know when changes occur and whether they are reactions to events or more persistent changes that signal a return of symptoms.

- After you've had more experience tracking your symptoms, you can use these graphs only when you suspect that your symptoms are returning. Monitor your mood or other prominent symptoms daily until they have stabilized.

- The effectiveness of medication changes can be monitored on a Mood or Symptom Graph. Begin tracking your mood as medications are added, decreased, or changed to determine the impact on your mood or other symptoms. Make notes on the graph as doses are changed to help you and your doctor monitor their effect.

- Mood and Symptom Graphs are helpful for communicating to your psychiatrist or therapist how you have been doing between visits, especially if they are separated by several weeks. Track your mood or symptoms daily and make notes on the graph about any circumstances you associate with improvements or worsening of your mood or symptoms. This will help you and your health care provider better understand your symptom fluctuations and what can be done to minimize the ones that are extreme or persistent.

- When you begin seeing a new doctor or therapist, you can help him or her get to know you and the pattern of your symptoms by monitoring your mood or other symptoms and taking the graphs to each visit. This will make it easier for you to communicate what happens between visits rather than having to rely solely on your memory.

Symptom Graph

The symptom I am tracking is:

Week of:	Plan	Sun	Mon	Tues	Wed	Thur	Fri	Sat
Manic +5	*Go to the hospital*	●	●	●	●	●	●	●
+4		●	●	●	●	●	●	●
+3	*Call the doctor*	●	●	●	●	●	●	●
+2	*Take action*	●	●	●	●	●	●	●
+1	*Watch closely*	●	●	●	●	●	●	●
0		●	●	●	●	●	●	●
−1	*Watch closely*	●	●	●	●	●	●	●
−2	*Take action*	●	●	●	●	●	●	●
−3	*Call the doctor*	●	●	●	●	●	●	●
−4		●	●	●	●	●	●	●
−5 **Depressed**	*Go to the hospital*	●	●	●	●	●	●	●

What caused the mood shift?

What's Next?

One of the goals of this book is to teach you ways to catch your mood swings when they are mild and easier to control. Some people are very aware of the subtle changes in their mood. They don't need the exercises in this chapter, but many others need help tracking the signs that depression or mania is starting. People tend to associate mood changes with the things and people around them rather than with their bipolar disorder. Use the exercises in this chapter to help you become aware of the signs. The next chapter will teach you about the common triggers that are associated with severe mood swings. Knowing more about how your mood fluctuates is a key to gaining more control over your mood swings.

5

Identify Triggers
and Improve Coping

In this chapter you will:

✓ Learn about common triggers for mood swings.

✓ Identify situations and events that may be triggering your mood swings.

✓ Become more aware of how you naturally cope when symptoms start.

✓ Find out about coping errors.

✓ Consider the role of medication in triggering and coping with mood swings.

Triggers

If you are like most people, you may be unaware of the things that set you off unless it's really obvious. As human beings, we react, positively and negatively, to events, people, situations, things we see or hear, or the stories that others tell us. The reaction can be quick, like a reflex, or take some time to evolve as we ponder, consider, or ruminate. With most things, the reaction ends when the event is over, like feeling frustrated when we can't find a parking space. Once we find a space, the negative feeling usually goes away. But sometimes events or triggers are big and the effect is lasting, or what starts as a small reaction can snowball into a more significant shift in your mood that is difficult to shake.

The goal of this chapter is to teach you about common triggers of mood swings that can persist or turn into episodes of depression, hypomania, or mania. If you know more about the kinds of things that might be associated with mood swings, you have a better chance of catching your symptoms as they begin to worsen. If you can do this, you have a better chance of taking action to keep them from turning into full episodes of depression or mania.

Another goal of this chapter is to make you more aware of how your reactions to triggers can make things better or can create bigger problems. Ideally, you want to be in control of your reactions; choose ways to cope that ease your discomfort rather than make things worse. Chapters 9 through 17 will help you strengthen your existing coping skills and teach you some new ones. This chapter helps prepare you by making you more aware of the ways you cope and ways in which your coping strategies could be improved.

Seasonal Mood Swings

Sometimes mood swings occur at predictable times. Common examples are depressions that occur during the winter months and manias that occur in the spring. In this case the shifting seasons can serve as triggers for mood swings. This is often referred to as a seasonal pattern or seasonal affective disorder (SAD). If you know that you are likely to have severe mood symptoms at a certain time of the year, you can prepare yourself and take precautions. For example, if you are likely to become manic in the spring, you might work with your doctor to monitor mood fluctuations more closely so that you can respond quickly if symptoms begin to emerge. You might also work with your psychiatrist to increase your dose of mood-stabilizing medications as a precaution. The same general strategy can be employed to help you avoid major depression in the winter months.

Maria says that she hates the holidays. On the one hand, she loves it when her family gets together at her grandmother's house for Christmas. Even thinking about the smell of tamales cooking in the kitchen can make her mouth water. On the other hand, her large family can get on her nerves. She has three older brothers, all married with children of their own. The kids are precious, but seeing them always leads to questions about when she will get married. She doesn't have the heart to tell her family that she doesn't want children or a husband. Maria's mother always makes a big deal out of buying and wrapping gifts, sending Christmas cards to family and friends, and cooking everyone's favorites. Maria doesn't have the energy to help with all of this, and she feels guilty about it every year. Since the Christmas holidays occur during the winter months, it is hard to know if Maria is being affected by seasonal changes or stresses related to holiday preparation. Perhaps it is the combination of both that affects her mood. In either case, recognizing the holidays as a potential trigger can help Maria plan for next year.

Stress

Stress is Raquel's trigger for mood swings—job stress is the biggest one. When she has too much to do and too little time to do it in, she gets overwhelmed and can't sleep. Depending on the season, Raquel can get depressed or manic. In the spring, missing sleep seems to make her more irritable and edgy, even if she is taking her meds consistently. In the winter, being overwhelmed can lead to self-criticism for her lack of productivity, lack of organizational ability, slowness, and mental confusion. This can make her feel depressed. Unfortunately, in her business, winter and spring tend to be the busiest times. Summers are slow, and she tends to have fewer symptom breakthroughs in the summer months. This may be a coincidence, it may reflect the fluctuation of her work stress, or it may result from a seasonal variation in her symptoms that makes her more vulnerable to day-to-day stresses at certain times of the year. It is hard to tell. Either way, Raquel has to put out more effort to control her symptoms in the early winter and the early spring than any other time of the year.

Relationship Events

Sometimes Paul's girlfriend, Angie, gets upset with him and will not return his calls. Sometimes it is Paul's fault for doing something stupid or inconsiderate, and sometimes it is Angie's fault because she overreacted to something small. Regardless of who started the conflict, not hearing from Angie really upsets him. At first he will get angry at her, but after a while he blames himself and feels depressed. What goes through Paul's mind is that Angie is one of the only girls who knows he is bipolar and accepts him as he is. She is special, and the thought of losing her is unbearable. Even when there is no conflict between Paul and Angie, he imagines the worst if she doesn't return his calls right away. The longer he has to wait, the more he blows the problem out of proportion, all the while knowing that he is probably overreacting. The fear of losing Angie is a big trigger for Paul's symptoms.

Sarah, Joe's wife, does not have bipolar disorder, but sometimes she feels really down, especially when her husband has done something to upset her. He has bipolar II disorder and a long history of alcohol abuse that has improved in recent years. They have been through a lot together, and she has stuck with him even when her friends advised her to leave him. The consequence is that she has very little tolerance for his hypomanic behavior, and any sign of it can trigger a bad mood for her. From Sarah's point of view, hypomania always leads to trouble for Joe and for their marriage. Last week he made a sexual joke in front of her mother, something he does only when he is having symptoms. Sarah immediately jumped all over him. When Joe denied being hypomanic and claimed he was just trying to make her laugh, she laid into him, bringing up all the other times his illness caused huge problems that were difficult to overcome. Joe is Sarah's trigger for mood swings.

Losses

The anniversary of a loss, such as the death of someone important in your life, can trigger significant mood swings. If this kind of trigger always gets you down, it may have something to do with how you cope with it and not just the fact that it occurred. Stan, Raquel's older brother, also has bipolar I disorder. He lost his best friend during the war in Iraq in 2003. Even after all these years, Stan can't bear to think about it. Around the anniversary of his friend's death, Stan starts detaching from others, drinks more, and gets high to dull his anger and his pain. If Raquel calls him, he just says, "I don't want to talk about it." A few times Raquel had to ask for a mental health warrant that led to Stan's hospitalization. When his depression and substance use lead to paranoia, the hospital is the only way she can get her brother back.

Tommy's parents split up when he was a kid. He had severe mood swings, but they didn't know what it was. They fought a lot about his behavior. Dad thought he needed discipline, and Mom thought he needed treatment. It took years to figure out that he had bipolar I disorder, and their marriage did not survive the stress. Eventually, Tommy got treated and his mother remarried. His real dad wanted nothing to do with Tommy, but luckily for Tommy, his stepfather really stepped up. Tommy was angry that his father had abandoned him, but he also felt guilty about his parents' marriage ending.

Like any married couple, Tommy's mother and stepfather occasionally had arguments, sometimes about how to handle Tommy. When he lived at home and overheard them, he felt a sense of panic when they fought that triggered a drop in his mood. He couldn't stand it, but he wasn't self-aware enough to understand how his reaction fed his depression. When times got particularly tough between his folks, he would get severely depressed and start talking about not wanting to live. This usually forced the attention back to him.

Sleep Changes

Sleep loss is a trigger for mania for lots of people who have bipolar I disorder. For Paul, it isn't always clear whether sleep loss triggers mania or mania makes him want to stay up all night. He is a very creative guy, and it is not unusual for him to get new ideas for projects while he is up late watching television. He is a software engineer with a new start-up company, and once he gets a new idea, he tends to want to work on it until it is done, while the creative juices are flowing. He gets so busy he often forgets to take his evening meds. By morning he is feeling wired and exhausted at the same time; his body wants to sleep, but his mind keeps going. So which came first—sleep loss, manic ideas, or forgetting his meds? It is never clear. What is important is that he recognizes the pattern and does something about it.

For people who tend to have more depression than mania or hypomania, sleep loss because of schedule changes, travel, a noisy environment, or feeling physically ill can lead to fatigue and lethargy that feel a lot like depression. Feeling sad can trigger upsetting thoughts, take away motivation, and reduce activity, which may snowball into a worsening mood.

Sentimental Things

Raquel is sentimental and gets tearful when watching commercials or when reminded of sad events. She was in church today when the priest talked about remembering those who died in war. She remembered her brother Stan's friend who had died in Iraq. Even though she had not thought about Charles in many years, she immediately began to cry. She remembered not only how sad she felt at the time, but how devastated Stan had been. She recalled the vacant look in the eyes of Charles's parents and imagined the pain they must still feel on days like this.

For Raquel, a sentimental or sad event like this can set the tone of her entire day. One sad thought makes her recall other sad events. She quickly draws associations between one sad memory and other sad memories, sad people, and sad moments. When she heard the music that marks the end of Sunday services, Raquel realized she had missed the whole thing, lost in her thoughts. On the walk home, she tried to tell herself to let it go, but it was too late. She had scheduled a day out with friends but was no longer in the mood to go. She stayed home, watched sad movies, worked her way through a half gallon of rocky road ice cream, and felt sorry for herself. She knew that she had a tendency to get like this—to do what she called "wallowing in misery." While part of her knew she needed to get over it before it snowballed, the other part of her found a strange comfort in it. Going out with friends and trying to be social was always a little uncomfortable for her. TV, ice cream, solitude, and sadness—this was what she knew how to do.

Positive Events

It is not only stressful or sad events that can trigger mood symptoms. Positive events can have the same effect if they lead to sleep loss, distract you from taking your medication regularly, or fool you into thinking that you are fine and don't need medication anymore. A good example is having a new baby. If you are a woman who had mood swings before giving birth, you will be more prone to new mood episodes after childbirth. If you are not the new mother but have a new child or a new puppy in your home, disruptions in your sleep can serve as the trigger for mood symptoms.

Not Addressing Your Problems

Some problems get resolved or go away with time. Others hang on and cause you stress when they recur or when you can't stop thinking about them. Maria, for example, thinks her boss discriminates against her because she is gay. He has never really said anything outright, but he definitely treats her differently than the other women in the office. To her face, one on one, he is respectful, but when they are at staff meetings, he occasionally talks to her in a hostile and condescending fashion, embarrassing her in front of others. From her experience, Maria knows that you can't accuse someone of discrimination without proof, so she has avoided talking to her boss about it. She tries to tell herself to shake it off, ignore him, or forgive him for his imperfections. But when he upsets her, she can't get it out of her head. She talks about it with her friends and family members and even some coworkers who have witnessed his outbursts. For weeks after an event, she finds that she thinks about it when she first wakes up in the morning, as she is trying to fall asleep at night, and even in church. And when she does, she feels angry all over again. She replays the event in her mind and adds in the things she wishes she had said to call him on it right then and there.

This is the kind of thing that triggers depression in Maria. She knows it, and she knows that not taking care of problems hurts her instead of the person who offended her. However, Maria also knows that it is hard to confront difficult problems and hurtful people, especially when there is reason to worry about the consequences of that confrontation. Maria wonders if she will get fired or if speaking up will just escalate her boss's disrespectful behavior. She likes her job, and she doesn't want to do anything to risk losing it. That is her dilemma.

Learn to Recognize Your Triggers

After you have been through a period of depression or mania, it's pretty common to try to look back and figure out what triggered the symptoms. It is hard to accurately remember when symptoms started unless it is something fairly obvious like discontinuing your medications or having a baby. Even stressful events like losing a job or ending a relationship may have been a consequence rather than the cause of mood swings. To learn more about your triggers, you will have to get some help from other people in your life and track your symptoms forward in time. In Chapter 4 you learned several strategies for monitoring your mood symptoms. You can use the same strategies to make note of the events that seemed to set them off.

It is not unusual to be able to remember things that triggered depression but not remember things that led to mania. That's why you will need help from family, friends, your doctor or therapist, or coworkers—anyone who was around you when your symptoms started. They may recall what was happening when your symptoms began even if you don't. Make notes in Exercise 5.1 on the next page of the types of events or situations that may have triggered your symptoms in the past.

Sometimes there are no obvious triggers for mood swings. You just wake up feeling bad. You might tell yourself that it is a premonition of bad things to come or that you woke up on the wrong side of the bed, had a bad dream, or got off on the wrong foot. Later in the day you might figure out what is bothering you, but sometimes there is no explanation. You could be just tired or hungry or starting to get physically ill, having hormone fluctuations, side effects from medications, seasonal allergies, or got a haircut you don't really like. Lots of things can set you off. Even if you can't pinpoint the trigger, you can learn to recognize the mood swings and do what you can to reduce your symptoms.

Coping Strategies

It is human nature to try to make yourself feel better when you are feeling bad. You try to get comfortable, calm yourself down, or perk yourself up. It is usually by trial and error that you figure out what works and what doesn't. You may have already figured out that there are things that can make you feel better, at least for a short while, but there are also some things that can actually make you feel worse. A good example is alcohol use. Some people turn to alcohol to reduce their anxiety, fall asleep at night, or feel more comfortable around others.

EXERCISE 5.1 Recognize Your Triggers		
In the spaces below, make some notes about the events you associate with the start of manic or depressive symptoms. Ask those who know you to help you fill in some examples.		
	Events that have triggered your depressive symptoms	**Events that have triggered your manic symptoms**
Seasonal		
Stressful events		
Relationship events		
Losses		
Sleep changes		
Sentimental things		
Positive events		

However, regular and/or excessive alcohol use can actually disrupt your sleep, make you say or do things that create new problems for you, or worsen your performance on the job. Soothing yourself with food is another common example. High-carbohydrate, high-sugar, and fatty foods can give you temporary comfort but may also lead to weight gain that makes you feel bad about yourself.

The next section has two goals. The first is to help you prepare for the next mood swing by learning to recognize positive and negative coping behaviors that you already use. The second goal is to help you develop new or make more use of existing coping strategies that have a better chance of reducing your symptoms without creating new problems along the way.

Things That Make You Feel Better

Most people are not aware of how their reactions to events are actually coping behaviors. For example, when Amanda is getting depressed, she sleeps, or at least pretends to be sleeping. When she is agitated or irritable, she lets off steam by yelling at her family members. While these are not ideal reactions, they do help her cope when she feels overwhelmed. At other times, Amanda goes to church to get support from her friends or sees her counselor.

Before she realizes it, Raquel reverts to basic coping strategies. She eats sweets to reduce stress or plays solitaire on her computer for hours on end instead of facing a problem. Avoidance works for her. Unfortunately, over the years she has put on an extra 80 pounds coping in this way. She hates herself for it, but not enough to learn new ways to cope. Raquel is learning to cope with bad feelings by leaving her physical space. She gets out of bed or off the couch, leaves her apartment, takes a shower, goes to the grocery store—anything that switches the focus away from her negative thoughts.

Joe drinks or gambles when he is feeling high and when he is feeling low. Miguel buys himself things. Tommy is new to bipolar disorder and doesn't know a lot about how it affects him. When he is feeling bad, he instinctively blames others for his problems. Although he may not call this a coping behavior, Tommy finds that running helps to burn off stress. It also helps him slow down, calms his racing thoughts, and makes him sleep better.

Paul hates being out of control, so he tries to be very consistent with his medications, but that doesn't always work. Stress, work, and seasonal changes still cause him to have occasional mood swings. Although he usually likes being around people, when he is feeling bad, he finds himself avoiding everyone. Sometimes this is a good coping strategy because it reduces stimulation and helps him avoid getting irritated when his family and girlfriend ask too many questions or try to "fix" him. It is a problem when he avoids them for too long and misses out on support or assistance that could pull him out of a slump.

All of these coping strategies work, albeit temporarily. They make the person feel better even if they do not permanently solve the problem. Take a moment and think about the things you do to soothe yourself. In Exercise 5.2 on the next page, make a list of things you are aware that you do to make yourself feel better. To make it easier, try to stick with recent situations. If you can't think of any, take some time to observe yourself during the next week or so. Pay attention to times when you don't feel right and watch what you do to cope. Then come back to Exercise 5.2 and make some notes about your coping behaviors.

Use Your Coping Resources

It is always easier to add a positive than to take away a negative when it comes to coping behaviors. For example, it is easier to start eating fruits and vegetables more often than it is to make yourself stop eating cookies. It is also easier to make use of your existing coping abilities than to create a new one. For example, it is easier to call someone you already know than to make a new friend.

Everyone possesses coping resources, even if they don't realize it. Personal qualities such as intelligence, a sense of humor, the ability to cook, or friendliness are all examples of coping resources. They help you make it through the day, overcome adversity, and deal with symptoms. Personal beliefs can also serve as coping resources, such as faith in God, belief in humanity, a strong work ethic, or ideas that drive you, like a desire to succeed, sense of responsibility to your family, or hope in the future.

EXERCISE 5.2   Coping Behaviors

Under the categories below, make note of some of the ways you have recently coped with feeling down, troubled, irritable, or high. Circle the ones that you rely on the most. Some examples have been provided.

Consuming things (e.g., comfort food, alcohol)

Distractions (e.g., television, Internet)

Substance use (e.g., smoking, drug use)

People (e.g., talking to or being around others)

Activity (e.g., exercise, cooking)

Avoidance or procrastination (e.g., staying in bed, avoiding people)

Self-expression (e.g., creativity, yelling)

Other coping behaviors

The people in your world can also be coping resources. Paul's girlfriend, Angie, for example, is a joy to be with and makes him feel good about himself. His parents, brothers, and nieces are all sources of support, and he seeks them out when he is feeling low. Maria has friends at work who make her laugh, and Amanda has friends at church who distract her from ruminating about her problems.

Activity is another type of coping resource. Paul enjoys sports; watching football and hockey on TV or attending games can lift his spirits except when his favorite team is losing to its biggest rivals. Raquel's brother Stan plays the piano to tune out upsetting thoughts. Tommy runs when he is agitated. Amanda cleans her house.

Seeking professional help is an obvious coping resource. Paul likes his psychiatrist, and Amanda trusts her counselor. In both cases, treatment strengthens their abilities to recognize symptoms as they are emerging, keep them from worsening, or push through periods of depression or mania.

In Exercise 5.3 below, make a list of coping resources that help you make it through your day, times of trouble, or periods when mood symptoms appear.

Change Your Environment

In the past, Amanda has walked off jobs when her anger and irritability hit a peak. For her, this is a symptom of hypomania or mania. Getting away from work was exactly what she needed, but waiting until she had a confrontation with a coworker or boss to do so usually resulted in her quitting her job or being terminated. Walking away from a fight, an argument, or an otherwise overstimulating environment is not a bad idea. The trick is in the timing.

Changing your environment can give you a moment to collect your thoughts, burn off some steam, calm down, and take time to think about what is happening to you. If it helps to reduce your emotions, you will be better able to reason things through and make good decisions. However, if you ignore the need to get away until you lose control, then your departure just creates a new problem. Although he has been sober for a few years, in the past Sarah would get irritated with Joe when he drank too much. He didn't listen to her when she asked him to stop, so she stopped asking. When he got obnoxious, she dropped the kids off at her mom's house and went shopping. They didn't have a lot of money, so she never really bought

---

EXERCISE 5.3	**What Are Your Coping Resources?**

Below are several categories of coping resources. Try to identify the resources you currently possess even if you do not use them on a regular basis.

Personal qualities that help me cope

My personal beliefs that keep me going

People who would provide support if I asked for it

Activities that give me some relief

Professionals who have helped me in the past

anything expensive. In fact, she didn't buy anything at all most of the time. Getting away from Joe, however, did her a world of good. After she shopped, she visited a friend or picked up the kids and took them to the movies—anything to avoid going home while he was drinking. For Sarah, changing environments didn't solve her husband's drinking problem, but it did help her cope and kept her from saying things that she might later regret.

A temporary change in environment can be helpful if it reduces overstimulation or irritation. Walking away from people who are causing you distress is also reasonable, as long as you do so before you blow up at them. A noisy household, restaurant, or mall may be more than you can handle when your concentration is poor or you are having racing thoughts. Excusing yourself from those situations can help you cope.

In the past, Joe would drink to change his environment, but this created marital problems, set a bad example for his kids, and made it hard for him to make it to work the next day. Getting intoxicated was one of his coping behaviors. It tuned out his stressful thoughts, worries, and problems and had the added benefit of causing his wife and kids to leave the house to avoid him. Quiet time to relax and take a break from his reality was what he really wanted. It took many years, the threat of losing his family, and some time in therapy before he learned this about himself. Now when he needs a change of environment to reduce his symptoms, he just tells his wife about it and they find a way to get him some time to himself.

A permanent change of environment may be called for if your current environment is making it hard for you to cope. This might include living with people who are opposed to psychiatric treatment, places where alcohol or drugs are hard to avoid, extremely stressful work environments, or locales that make you more prone to seasonal affective disorder or where mental health treatment is not available.

Strengthen Your Healthy Habits

If you are like most people, you probably use a mix of healthy and unhealthy coping strategies. Unhealthy coping is usually quick, easy, and brings instant, albeit temporary, relief. Coping in a healthy way can create more lasting effects. What feels like quick relief is what makes most people impulsively use poor coping strategies. It is not that they work better. They just seem to work better. To make changes in your coping habits you will need to convince yourself that it is worth the effort.

Go back to Exercise 5.2 on page 66, where you listed commonly used coping behaviors, and pick a negative one that you think may be worth changing or a positive one that you think you should use more often. Use the next exercise (Exercise 5.4 on the facing page) to consider the advantages and disadvantages of making this change.

Make a Plan to Improve Your Coping Skills

The first few chapters of this book are intended to help you better understand your mood swings, what triggers them, and how you normally respond. In the chapters that follow, you will learn a number of new skills for controlling your symptoms. If you have been living with

EXERCISE 5.4 Why Change My Coping Behaviors?
Select one coping behavior from Exercise 5.2 to either increase or decrease. Think about the advantages and the disadvantages of changing this coping behavior.
I would like to reduce my use of the following coping behavior:
I would like to increase my use of the following coping behavior: What are the advantages of making this change? How will it help you? What will be difficult about making this change?

MARIA'S EXAMPLE Why Change My Coping Behaviors?
I would like to increase my use of the following coping behavior: *I would like to tell people when they have offended me instead of avoid it.* What are the advantages of making this change? How will it help you? What will be difficult about making this change? *It is better to speak up about it. When I say nothing, it lets the person get away with being rude. I need to stick up for myself. I can't expect them to read my mind. It is not easy, because I don't know what kind of reaction I will get.*

mood swings for some time, you have probably already found a number of ways to cope—some good and some not so helpful. This chapter has focused on helping you identify the ways you naturally cope so that you can make conscious decisions to use strategies that are effective and reduce your reliance on strategies that give you only short-term relief from discomfort. Use Exercise 5.5 on the next page to set some goals for strengthening your coping abilities. Practice these methods between mood episodes so that they can be well learned and automatic when you need them to cope with depression or mania. As you continue to work your way through this book, you will add to your coping resources and begin to more effectively manage your symptoms.

EXERCISE 5.5   Strengthen Your Coping Skills

For each heading, set a goal for how you might be able to use this strategy more often to help you cope with your mood swings.

Use Your Coping Resources (which ones?)

Change Your Environment (when would it help?)

Avoid Self-Defeating Behaviors (what would you do instead?)

Strengthen Your Healthy Habits (what habits do you already have?)

What's Next?

This chapter introduced you to common triggers that can set off mood swings. You can combine this new information with the exercises you did in Chapter 4 to help you begin to create an early warning system that lets you catch symptoms before you feel out of control. You also learned about some simple strategies for coping with mood swings. They can help you begin to regain some control when you feel like your symptoms are worsening. The next chapter will add to these new skills by drawing your attention to common things that can make you feel worse rather than better. If you can avoid making things worse, you will have a chance to improve your mood symptoms by using the skills presented in the remaining chapters of this workbook.

Step 3

Don't Make It Worse

6

Avoid Things
That Make You Feel Worse

In this chapter you will:

✓ Learn about things you do that might worsen your mood.

✓ Identify things you say to yourself that can make your symptoms worse.

✓ Discover new ways to deal with hopeless and suicidal thoughts.

There are things you can do to make yourself feel better, but there are also many things you can do to make your symptoms worse. For example, when you are feeling blue, watching movies with tragic themes, listening to sad songs, or thinking about past losses can feed your depression. Your low mood might make you gravitate toward these things, but exposing yourself to them will only make you feel worse.

Similarly, if you are feeling irritable, going to places that are noisy and crowded, watching television news, or being around people with negative attitudes can make you feel crankier. You might tell yourself, "I'm already in a bad mood, so what difference will it make?" But if you want to feel better, you can start by figuring out how not to make your mood worse.

In this chapter, you will learn about common thoughts and actions that can worsen symptoms of bipolar disorder. Some may sound familiar to you, and others may be behaviors or ideas you've never associated with mood swings. For example, when some people enter an up or manic phase, they often crave nighttime activity and stimulation, but these things can make their symptoms more intense and harder to control. That's because losing nighttime sleep can escalate hypomania and mania. Even if you try to take naps to compensate for sleep loss, disruptions in your normal sleep–wake cycle have been shown to make mood swings worse.

When you are able to detect the early signs of a mood swing (see Chapters 3 and 4), your next order of business should be to not make them worse. As you read through the examples in this chapter, make a list of things you want to try to avoid or habits you want to try to break. Add them to your plan to gain control of your mood swings.

What You Say to Yourself That Can Make Mood Swings Worse

It is human nature to talk ourselves into things. When we are feeling good, we can convince ourselves that everything will be OK or that our favorite sports teams are going to win. When we are in a bad mood, we can convince ourselves that we are destined to fail or that there is nothing we can do to help ourselves when faced with tough situations. We are very good at persuading ourselves even when there is no real evidence to support our ideas. We trust our gut instincts or feelings because sometimes we are right.

Unfortunately, this tendency can make things worse when it works against efforts to control your mood symptoms. Below are some things that people say to themselves when they are faced with making decisions about managing their mood disorders such as bipolar disorder. If any of them are things you have said to yourself, think about how these ideas might interfere with your goal of controlling your mood swings. Make an effort to reason through counterproductive thoughts rather than relying on your feelings to guide you.

"I Don't Have a Mental Illness."

If you have had the unpleasant experience of being given bad news such as a diagnosis of bipolar disorder, then you are probably familiar with the feeling of resisting an idea. A diagnosis of a chronic mental illness is hard to hear, even if you think it is correct. It is natural to psychologically and emotionally push it away, even after years of living with the illness and receiving treatment for it. This is usually called denial, and it tends to make matters worse.

Denial is a normal coping response when we receive information that is emotionally and psychologically unacceptable. Denial protects us from the discomfort that comes with having to accept something unpleasant, painful, or inconsistent with how we think about ourselves. It is denial that is operating when you can't sleep and you look exhausted but you tell people, "I'm fine. No, really, I'm fine." When your mood is highly irritable and you feel agitated and have racing thoughts, denial is doing its job when you tell yourself, "It's not me. Everyone else is just getting on my nerves." When you know that you need medication to resolve your depression, but you don't want to take it, you use denial to convince yourself that you are feeling better and that the episode "will pass."

Denial usually operates unconsciously. Because you may not realize that you are doing it, it can be hard to fix. To keep denial in check, listen to your own words when you talk about your mood symptoms. When you feel bad but tell others that you are "OK," you are denying that you have a problem. While you may deny feeling bad to try to reduce your family members' worry, you are also trying to persuade yourself that nothing is wrong. Rather than resist the idea that you are having mood symptoms, follow your doctor's treatment advice and learn new skills to control mood swings. If you think you may be in denial about your mood swings, the exercises in Chapter 12 might help you learn more about how to ease into acceptance.

"I'm Tired of Trying."

The low energy, loss of motivation, mental slowness, and hopelessness that are brought about by depression can also convince you that you would be better off if you didn't take medicine, stopped going to doctors, and gave up on the endless struggle to control your illness. The effort it takes to manage your illness can leave you mentally and emotionally exhausted at times. To cope with these feelings, some people take breaks from trying to control their illness. For a few days they feel a sense of freedom, but unfortunately, this usually makes matters worse.

Wanting to give up because you're tired of trying is a normal feeling. People feel that way when they are tired of their jobs, tired of school, tired of taking care of small children, tired of trying to get out of debt, and tired of trying to find the right partner. If you're facing these kinds of life struggles along with trying to control your illness, you have the right to be especially exhausted. Life can be very hard. To cope with these times, you have to add positives to your life to balance out all the negatives. If you have some good things to look forward to, people who give you pleasure or make you smile, reasons to rush home after a long day at work, these things will help you hang in there and put out the effort to be at your best. If you lack positives in your life, it's time to add them. A few examples are provided in Chapter 15, but use your imagination to make your life worth the effort it takes to stay well.

If you are tired of trying because you are not getting what you need out of medication treatment or psychotherapy, rather than giving up, perhaps you should consider making a change. Start by sharing your concerns with your clinician before you stop any treatments on your own. Keep in mind that stopping medications suddenly can put you at risk for a relapse. If you have worked with your clinician and are still unsatisfied, it may be time to get another opinion.

It's Time to Make a Change

It is normal to want change in your life from time to time. We all get the urge to change our hairstyle, move to a new place, repaint our house, rearrange our furniture, learn a new hobby, change jobs, or otherwise make our lives more interesting. Most of the time there is nothing wrong with change. It can become a negative, however, if too many changes are attempted at the same time or if those changes are not well thought out and lead to bigger problems.

Mood swings that are associated with hypomania or mania often include a flood of new ideas and impulsivity—the tendency to act before thinking. When reasoning is colored by an up mood, dramatic changes such as quitting your job, having an affair, or buying something expensive can all seem reasonable and justified. However, giving in to a big urge can make matters worse.

Create Emotional Distance

One strategy for coping with the urge to change is to put some time between having an idea for change and taking action on it. During that pause you have time to think through the change you are considering, consider the pros and cons, and make a decision that is best for you. Exercise 6.1 (below) includes some questions you might consider when you feel the urge to make a major change in your life.

The 24-Hour Rule

The 24-hour rule is an agreement that you make with yourself or with the important people in your life to hold off 24 hours on making decisions or taking actions that involve doing something that you would not normally do, that others would object to, or that may involve some risks. If something is a good idea today, it will be a good idea tomorrow, so a 24-hour delay should not cause any harm. The 24-hour delay gives you time to use the other methods in this workbook to sort through your thoughts so that when you make a decision to act, it will not be something you later regret. If 24 hours is not enough time, make it a 48-hour rule. Tommy uses the 24-hour rule before he gives in to his urge to travel. Raquel uses the 24-hour rule when she gets the urge to overspend at the mall. Amanda uses the 24-hour rule before scolding her husband. She figures if an issue is worth risking marital conflict over, it

EXERCISE 6.1 Is Change a Good Idea?
Use your reasoning ability and/or ask people you trust to help you respond to the questions below about the major change you are considering. Think carefully about the answers before you take action.
• Do I really want to make this change?
• Is it worth my time and energy?
• How much effort am I willing to put out?
• Does anyone else think this is a good idea?
• Am I having a general urge for change, or am I really dissatisfied with how things are?

will still be important the next day. If she gives herself 24 hours to cool off, she is more likely to handle the situation with tact instead of biting her husband's head off.

Make a Small Change

If you believe the desire for change is driven by hypomania or mania, another strategy is to take the necessary precautions to control symptoms and then ask yourself if there is something small you can change to satisfy the need. Instead of buying a new car, can you wash and wax the one you have? Instead of moving to a new apartment, is there something you can change in your old one that will make it more attractive or better organized? Can you rearrange things to make more space rather than getting a bigger place? If you have the urge to change your hair color, pick a temporary coloring product that will wash out if you change your mind. Rather than getting an extreme haircut, try styling it differently or ask a friend or hair specialist to do it for you. If you want a new look, work with the clothes you have rather than buying new things. If you need accessories, go to a discount or resale store before spending money on purchases you might later regret. If you want to make bigger changes, such as in boyfriends, girlfriends, lovers, or spouses, read Chapter 16 on effective decision making first.

Actions That Make Mood Swings Worse

Skipping Medication

Not taking medication can make things worse. Even skipping a few doses can be harmful because it lowers the amount of the drug in your system, making it ineffective. For some, discontinuing the use of medications for a short time can be a type of personal protest, but the only person it harms is you.

If you're not convinced that you need to stay on medication or if you think your regimen needs to change, talk it over with your doctor before you take any action. Remember that the symptoms of bipolar disorder can alter your thinking and make you feel discouraged about taking medication. Take time to evaluate your thoughts before making any dramatic changes.

Staying High

The enjoyment of highs—positive mood swings—before they get out of control is the reason some people try to extend them. Their hope is to stay hypomanic without letting it become a full episode of mania. Unfortunately, it rarely works out that way. Hypomania can easily evolve into mania for people with bipolar I disorder. Although most would say that in the long run it's not worth the risk, trying to ride out the high is still one of the common things people do that inevitably make matters worse.

Most people are able to think logically when they are hypomanic even when their symptoms are pushing them to act impulsively. It may be difficult to ignore the urge to stay high, but there is often another part of you that doesn't want to suffer the consequences that mania can bring. To keep yourself from making things worse when your mood is up, you should consider creating a plan for what to do the next time it happens. The plan can be as simple as writing a note reminding yourself about how hypomania affects you and the consequences you may face if you don't do what you can to rein in it. Keep the note in a handy place, like on your bulletin board, smartphone, or computer desktop so you won't have to hunt for it when you need it.

Tommy has had some significant manic episodes, so he thought he would give this exercise a try. Below is his note that he wrote on an index card and taped to his bedroom mirror frame at about eye level. After reading Tommy's example, create a plan of your own in Exercise 6.2 on the facing page.

Follow Tommy's example and create a plan in Exercise 6.2 for what to do if you feel like you are getting high or manic. Make a copy of the plan and put it in a convenient place or give it to someone you trust. Worksheets like this work only if you can find them when you need them and if the ideas are your own. Give it a try!

Losing Sleep

Losing the ability to sleep is a symptom of hypomania and mania, but it is also what seems to make the problem worse. Studies on sleep patterns in mood disorders have shown that loss of sleep can push a person with bipolar disorder into mania. Sleep loss can be caused by travel, thinking about problems at bedtime, working overtime, hearing disturbing noises at night, or getting too involved in fun activities around bedtime. Losing sleep for these reasons

---

TOMMY'S EXAMPLE   **What I Need to Remember about the Risks of Staying High**

What to Do If I Want to Stay High

by Tommy

You've been here before. Don't go there again.

Living out the highs is a fantasy with a dark side.

It lies to you, seduces you, and tries to convince you that it's safe.

BUT IT'S NOT!

The highs lead to the hospital and to humiliation. Don't go there.

Remember that there are ways to feel good and to have fun without the risks of mania.

You've been there before. Don't go there again.

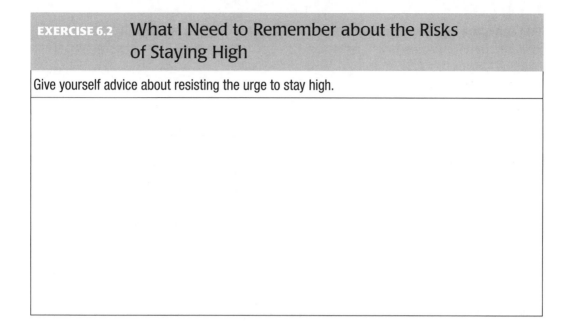

can quickly turn into insomnia, in which you can't fall asleep. Most sleep researchers suggest going to bed and waking up at about the same time each day. To prevent your symptoms from worsening, follow these simple rules: Avoid all-nighters, schedule travel to ensure a good night's sleep, and work out your worries before you go to bed.

Anger

If you have been through periods of depression in the past, it's easy to get angry with yourself when symptoms return. But getting angry about being depressed only makes you feel worse. Getting depressed about the fact that you're going through another episode of depression compounds your misery, making it harder to bring yourself out of the episode. It's OK to be angry about having bipolar disorder and being forced to go through another round of depression. You have the right to be mad, frustrated, or disappointed. However, it's best to acknowledge your annoyance and then let it go long enough to work at pulling yourself through it. Staying mad only fuels the fire.

Make a Self-Protection Plan

Keeping yourself from making things worse takes some planning. You have to know what worsens your mood swings and make a commitment to avoid those things the next time you are feeling too high or too low, and you need a reminder of what to avoid and how to avoid it. Use Exercise 6.3 (p. 80) to begin creating your Self-Protection Plan. Start by making a list of the things you know can worsen your depression or mania and note what you will do about

My Self-Protection Plan

Things that can make my depression worse	What I am going to do about it

Things that can make my mania worse	What I am going to do about it

them the next time your symptoms worsen. Include any examples described in this chapter that sound like you. If you are not sure what worsens your mood swings, ask a family member, a friend, or your doctor or therapist to help you come up with ideas. Those who know you well can probably tell you about the last time your mood went from bad to worse.

It has been a long time since Raquel has had a full manic episode, but she does get mildly manic or hypomanic from time to time. Below are her ideas for keeping her symptoms from worsening when they appear.

Considering Suicide

There may be times when thoughts about death or suicide might seem reasonable or feel comforting. Severe depression can darken your thinking to such a degree that you might be able to convince yourself that dying is your only option. These are scary thoughts that often lead to hurtful acts against yourself in an attempt to take your own life. Allowing yourself to

RAQUEL'S EXAMPLE My Self-Protection Plan	
Things that can make my depression worse	**What I am going to do about it**
Thinking about the past Listing my faults and failures	Cook a meal to distract myself Think about my children
Watching sad movies on TV	Get out of bed, turn off TV, and do something in another room
Getting "advice" from my mom	Screen my calls; call her when I'm feeling better
Drinking wine	Don't buy it when feeling down
Things that can make my mania worse	**What I am going to do about it**
Shopping in malls, especially during big sales	Avoid them when manic or limit shopping to necessities
Surfing the Internet late at night	Check e-mail in the morning or get online right after dinner
Family gatherings—too many people and too much noise	Don't go or leave early
Staying up all night to watch TV	Read in bed instead of watching TV

spend a lot of time thinking about suicide usually makes your mood worse and puts you at higher risk of acting on your impulses.

Suicidal thoughts can take many forms. In their most severe form, you might hear voices instructing you to kill yourself. These are auditory hallucinations, triggered by the biological changes occurring in your brain when you are depressed. They are not your true thoughts. A milder form of suicidal thoughts might include vague ideas about dying or a desire to just run away or disappear. In the middle range, there might be thoughts that it would be OK with you if your death occurred, although you wouldn't necessarily do anything to bring it about. Some people wish they could fall asleep peacefully and not wake up.

Thoughts about death or suicide are usually the result of feeling hopeless about the future and helpless to make anything change. When you can't think of any other solutions to your problems and can see no reason to hold on, death may begin to seem like an acceptable option. But it's not your only option.

Caution!

- Fantasies about suicide can be very **seductive**. They can trick you into thinking that death will be better than life.
- Fantasies about suicide can give you **false comfort**. They can fool you into believing that death is the reasonable solution to your problems.
- Fantasies about suicide **delude you** into thinking that no one will mind. They allow you to conjure up fake images of everyone being better off without you. They do not allow you to see the grief and misery you will leave behind. They keep you from imagining the guilt that will plague your family and friends for not having saved you.
- Fantasies are not only dangerous for you; they **set a dangerous standard** for others. Children who have a parent who has committed suicide are more likely to commit suicide themselves. Suicide can mean condemning those who love you to a similar fate.

What to Do When You Have Thoughts about Suicide

Do not wait until the last minute to ask for help. If you find that you have active thoughts about killing yourself or less specific ideas that death would be all right with you, tell someone about it. Tell a family member, call your doctor or therapist, or ask a member of the clergy for help. Do not trust yourself to set limits on your suicidal fantasies.

Get help if you experience any of the following:

- Thoughts about suicide, including fantasies about how you might do it
- Recurrent thoughts about death in general
- Envy for people who are dead or who are dying
- Giving away your possessions
- Hearing yourself saying good-bye to family members, friends, or pets
- Beginning to prepare people to live without you

- Becoming aware of things in your environment that can help you commit suicide
- Starting to hoard your medication so you will have enough for an overdose
- Viewing warning labels as prescriptions for suicide

The goal of this workbook is to teach you ways to prevent or reduce your symptoms of depression and mania before they get out of control, in this case, before they get to the point that suicide starts to be an attractive idea. If you use the exercises for monitoring your mood changes, are as consistent as you can be with your medication, and learn the methods presented so far for controlling your symptoms, you can stop episodes of depression and mania from getting out of control.

Reasons to Live

To have a chance to change your life for the better, you have to stick around long enough to learn something new. Try doing Exercise 6.4 at the bottom of this page to help yourself fight off thoughts about death and dying. List your reasons to live. Plan ahead for times when you might have doubts that life is worth living. List things you would want to remind yourself of when times are bad. You may download and print additional copies of this exercise from *www.guilford.com/basco2-forms* and add them to your workbook as needed.

EXERCISE 6.4 Reasons to Live

Make a list of reasons to continue living. When you begin to have dark thoughts about life, look over the list to remind yourself of these reasons so you can hold on for another day.

Reasons I shouldn't leave:

People to live for:

Things I would miss:

Experiences I have not yet had:

Things that matter to me:

From *The Bipolar Workbook, Second Edition.* Copyright 2015 by The Guilford Press.

PAUL'S EXAMPLE Reasons to Live

Reasons I shouldn't leave:

There are things I want to do with my life.
I'm not a quitter.

People to live for:

My mom, my grandmother, my girlfriend, my best friend, my nieces, my brother

Things I would miss:

Hockey games, the Super Bowl, sausage pizza, sex

Experiences I have not yet had:

I want to buy a new car.
I want to see the Grand Canyon.
I want to learn to scuba dive.

Things that matter to me:

My family and Angie

Paul went through a few serious bouts of depression and even tried to kill himself with an overdose of pills. He remembers working his way out of wanting to die by thinking of reasons to stick around. Above is an example of Paul's list of reasons to live. It will give you an idea of how to create your own plan.

Reasons to Have Hope

When you feel depressed enough to have suicidal thoughts, you might think there is no other way to solve your problems. You may have temporarily lost confidence in your ability to pull out of the slump you're in. When others try to encourage you or express their confidence in your ability to get better, you might minimize it because it does not fit with your negative view at the time. There may be good reasons to be hopeful about the future, but the tunnel vision that clouds your thinking when you are severely depressed does not let you see them. Because of this, it's best to make your list of reasons to have hope at a time when you are feeling more confident and hopeful. When you're depressed, you can read the list to remind yourself that your outlook can be more positive and that part of you knows there are reasons to be hopeful. In Exercise 6.5 on the facing page, make a list of reasons that you believe there might be hope for your future. You may download and print additional copies of this exercise from *www.guilford.com/basco2-forms* and add them to your workbook as needed.

EXERCISE 6.5 Reasons to Have Hope

Make a list of reasons to have hope. The following questions might help.

- What are you currently doing that gives you hope for improvement?

- Is it possible that the problems that bring you down are only temporary?

- Have you made it through difficult times in the past?

- Why do other people believe there is hope for your future?

- When you are not depressed, what kinds of things give you hope?

AMANDA'S EXAMPLE Reasons to Have Hope

My Reasons for Hope:

I have a lot of people in my life who love me and help me through difficult times.

I have gotten depressed and lost hope before, but I have also gotten it back.

I am a strong person. If I can survive childbirth, I can survive this.

I always think this way when I'm depressed. It will pass.

I have a good doctor and a good therapist who will help me survive.

My kids are my reason for hope.

I just started on a new medication that the doctor thinks will pull me out of this.

I know there is more I can do to help myself.

Review your list from time to time and add new reasons you can think of to be hopeful. Keep the list where you will be able to find it when you start to doubt that life is worth living.

Clinicians take even your most vague thoughts of suicide seriously, and so should you. They know that a general notion that life may not be worth living or that you would like to go to sleep and never wake up could turn into an active plan to commit suicide. Sometimes clinicians, family members, and friends may seem to overreact when you make comments that suggest that death is on your mind. They overreact because they don't know how close you are to acting on these ideas. While you may take comfort in thoughts about death, they feel a sense of panic and responsibility for your well-being. They don't want to lose you even if in those moments you are not worried about losing them.

What's Next?

It is instinctual to try to make yourself feel better when you are having symptoms of bipolar disorder. Unfortunately, without realizing it you can sometimes make matters worse rather than better. This chapter covered several situations, activities, and responses that may make your symptoms of depression and mania worse. The goal was to increase your awareness of them so that you can avoid or stop them when you realize what is happening. The same theme carries over to the next chapter, where you will learn how your thought patterns can make your symptoms worse. You will begin to learn skills for controlling thoughts that feed your emotions. The idea is for you to switch your coping strategies from things that may be instinctual, but not helpful, to things that make you feel better.

7

Don't Let Your Emotions Control Your Thoughts

In this chapter you will:

✓ Find out how your mood affects your thoughts.

✓ Discover the connection between your mood and your actions.

✓ Uncover new ways to keep yourself from overreacting.

Many people who live with recurring mood swings, such as those with bipolar disorder, often complain that they feel like their emotions are controlling their lives. They feel helpless, as if they have no control over the mood swings that dominate their lives. In this chapter, you will learn how your mood swings influence your thoughts and choice of actions and what you can do about it.

Thoughts and Feelings

By this point in the workbook you have probably figured out that the strategies for controlling your mood swings center around the connection between your mood, actions, and thoughts. In the sections that follow, the connection between thoughts and feelings will be described more fully. What you may find out is that you have more control over your emotions than you previously thought. Knowing how your thoughts, feelings, and actions influence each other will give you the freedom to make different choices on how to cope.

Your Mood Has a Strong Influence on Your Attitude

Have you ever noticed that when you are in a bad mood your outlook on life is negative? You are more self-critical, your outlook on the future seems bleak, and the world seems to be full of hardship and little hope? You might have some of the same views on a good day, but when you are having a bad day it is easier to focus and dwell on the negatives. This is because your mood greatly influences your view of yourself, the future, other people, and the world.

If you have positive changes in your mood or experience euphoria that comes with hypomania and mania, you may notice that a positive mood makes you view yourself in an overly positive light. Your confidence may grow, your opportunities may seem limitless, and the people around you may seem to find you more attractive and interesting. If you are like many people with a bipolar spectrum disorder and your euphoria switches into irritability, you probably know firsthand how those positive thoughts can quickly darken. You may continue to think well of yourself, but you begin to see other people as interfering with your life, stupid, or controlling. Once your mood returns to normal you may not remember these dramatic changes in your attitude or you may believe that they were logical thoughts given the circumstances at the time.

Your Mood Can Also Strongly Influence Your Choice of Actions

When your mood swings and attitude are strong enough, they can have an influence on your choice of actions. For example, an irritable mood and a negative outlook on others can make you snap at others, such as your children or your coworkers, because they seem to be bothering you. An anxious mood and a fearful outlook can keep you from getting information or solving problems because you anticipate a bad outcome. A euphoric mood and a fearless outlook can lead you to take unnecessary risks because you think nothing can go wrong. These are all examples of how your mood can control your choice of actions. Other common examples include isolating yourself from others, acting without thinking, poor decision making, buying things you can't afford, and self-medicating with alcohol or street drugs.

Mood Swings Can Make You Overreact

Bipolar disorder produces strong emotions such as sadness, irritability, excitement, anxiety, and anger during episodes of depression and mania and sometimes between episodes as well. These emotions or mood swings can make you more prone to overreact to upsetting situations. For example, when Amanda is depressed, she is more easily overwhelmed when there is too much to do. Last week Amanda's son told her on Sunday afternoon that he had a project due at school the next morning and he needed some supplies from the store. Amanda already had plenty of chores to do that day and resented this last-minute announcement. When she found out that the assignment had been given 2 weeks before, she could feel her blood boil. Even though her son was just a middle schooler, she got angry and complained that he was irresponsible, inconsiderate, and unappreciative of how hard she works. He apologized and went to his room. After she calmed down, she felt bad about yelling at him, so she put aside her chores, took him to the store, and helped him with his project. When Amanda is not depressed, she still doesn't like things to upset her schedule, but she doesn't usually overreact and yell at her kids over small things.

Have you ever found yourself feeling overwhelmed? Look at Amanda's example below and then take a moment and write down in Exercise 7.1A a recent event that upset you, the thoughts that went through your head, and how you reacted to the situation.

Your mood swings set you up to overreact, but what determines your response to events is what you think about the situation. Amanda was in a bad mood to start with, but the reason she reacted so strongly to her son was that she thought his request meant that he did not value her time and how hard she worked. At that moment, she thought that if he valued her time he would not drop things on her at the last minute. In this situation Amanda thought

AMANDA'S EXAMPLE Events, Thoughts, and Actions— Feeling Overwhelmed		
Amanda's trigger event	**Amanda's thoughts**	**How Amanda handled it**
Amanda's son told her at the last minute that he had a project to do.	*He's irresponsible. He is inconsiderate. He does not appreciate how hard I work and how much I have to do.*	Yelled at her son and made him feel bad. Later felt bad. Took him to the store and helped him with his project.

EXERCISE 7.1A Events, Thoughts, and Actions— Feeling Overwhelmed		
Your trigger event	**Your thoughts**	**How you handled it**

the issue was about her when it was actually about a kid who forgot to do his homework project.

It's easy to see how external events can trigger an emotional reaction like the one Amanda had toward her son. What you may know from experience is that the emotional changes that occur during periods of depression and mania can stir up emotional thoughts even when nothing in particular is happening. Here is another example from Amanda.

Amanda's depression makes her feel down and doubt that things will ever get better. The more she thinks about her problems, the more hopeless she feels. She says things to herself like "I can't believe my life is such a mess. I'm never going to get out of debt. I can't keep up with this house and the kids and my job. I may as well just give up." If she starts thinking this way when she wakes up in the morning, she feels no motivation to get out of bed, to interact with the family, or to pay her bills, even though she knows they are overdue. Amanda's depression affects her thoughts, making them negative and hopeless. Both her bad mood and her dark thoughts take away her motivation to get up and take on another day. She stays in bed, lets her husband tend to the kids, and leaves the bills on her desk for another day.

Amanda's examples have shown how your mood can affect your thoughts and your choice of actions during periods of depression, but the same thing can happen during periods of elevated mood. During his last two manic episodes, Tommy felt euphoric for a while but later became irritable and angry. Here is an example of the type of thing that would occur.

Tommy was feeling edgy when he walked into his parents' house to have dinner with them. His mother noticed that Tommy was pacing around a lot more than usual and asked him if he had taken his medication. Tommy blew up at her. "Get off my case about the medicine. I hate taking that stuff. You're always badgering me about it. Why do you have to make me angry? Can't we get through one evening without you bringing that up again? I'm leaving." Tommy went out the door and slammed it behind him, got in his car, and sped away. He went to a friend's house and drank a few beers until he calmed down enough to go back to his apartment. Have you ever had experiences like this? Take a moment to write down in Exercise 7.1B an example of how irritability makes you overreact.

As with depression, mania can produce spontaneous thoughts that arouse emotions, like suddenly getting a great idea and feeling really good about it. Spontaneous creative

TOMMY'S EXAMPLE Events, Thoughts, and Actions—Irritability		
Tommy's trigger event	**Tommy's thoughts**	**How Tommy handled it**
His mom asked him if he had taken his medication.	*She's on my case. She is badgering me. She knows I hate taking medications and she still brings it up.*	Yelled at his mom. Left without eating dinner. Sped off in his car. Drank beer until he could calm down.

EXERCISE 7.1B Events, Thoughts, and Actions—Irritability		
Your trigger event	**Your thoughts**	**How you handled it**

thoughts or ideas can be very exciting and make you want to pursue them even if it isn't practical at the time. Paul is generally a very creative person. When he is in the beginning of a hypomanic or manic episode, he often experiences what feels like a flood of creative ideas. For example, he was up late watching television because he couldn't fall asleep. He saw a commercial about a new reading program for kids who had difficulty in school. He was thinking about being a kid and having a lot of trouble with reading when a wonderful idea came to mind for a program that would be so much better than the one in the commercial. Paul went to his computer to write down his ideas. At 3:00 A.M. Paul noticed that he was getting tired and remembered that he had to be at work by 8:00 A.M. He knew himself fairly well and realized that for the last 3 hours he had been experiencing a manic burst of energy. He knew that if he stayed up all night and worked on his project his mania could get worse. He looked at the pillbox sitting on his nightstand and realized that he had not taken his medication earlier. Taking it now would make him sleep through the alarm, so he turned off the computer and tried to sleep without it. After tossing and turning for some time he was able to fall asleep for a few hours before the alarm went off.

Paul's new idea may have been an excellent one and worthy of his time. The problem was not the project. The problem was the timing. Going with his spontaneous idea made him forget his evening medication and kept him up much later than he could afford. The end result was that the next day Paul was exhausted at work, but his mind was beginning to race, another symptom that mania was coming.

Think of a time when you might have had an experience like Paul's and write about it in Exercise 7.1C on the next page. Try to remember how you felt compelled to take action right away rather than wait for a time that was more convenient. Mania can make you think that things are more urgent than they really are and that if you don't take action right away you will lose your wonderful idea altogether. The actions taken can create new problems if they disrupt your sleep and make you forget to take your medication.

PAUL'S EXAMPLE Events, Thoughts, and Actions—Hypomania		
Paul's trigger event	**Paul's thoughts**	**How Paul handled it**
Sees a TV commercial that stimulates a creative idea about a reading program	*I have a great idea. It's so much better than the one on TV. I better work on it right now, before I lose the idea. This is going to make me a lot of money.*	Got out of bed. Didn't take his evening medications. Worked at the computer until 3:00 A.M. Slept for only a few hours before having to go to work.

EXERCISE 7.1C Events, Thoughts, and Actions—Hypomania		
Your trigger event	**Your thoughts**	**How you handled it**

Each of the examples provided shows how emotions can set you up to overreact to internal or external events. Your reactions are based on your evaluation of the situation—that is, what you think about it. As illustrated, the thoughts fueled by depression or mania can be distorted by emotions. They can be overly negative or overly positive, depending on your mood. The bigger problem is that your emotional reactions and what you think about a situation will dictate how well you handle it. If you're not seeing things accurately, you're not always going to handle the situation well.

Thinking Errors

The exercises in this next section are aimed at helping you recognize when your mood is distorting your perceptions and causing you to overreact. If you can catch overly emotional

thoughts when they occur, you can take control of them rather than letting them control your reactions. One way to do this is to try to become aware of when you are thinking in an overly emotional way. If you can catch it happening, you have a chance to control it by using your logic and by choosing a good course of action.

To catch distorted thinking you have to know what to look for. There are some common patterns in the ways depression and mania can color your thinking. They are called thinking errors. The following sections describe some of the more common thinking errors people make when depressed and when manic. If you can catch yourself making any of these thinking errors, you will have an opportunity to correct the distortions before they lead you in the wrong direction.

One of the most common mistakes that people make is jumping to conclusions before they have all the information they need to fully understand a situation. You can jump to conclusions by making guesses or assumptions about people or about events. In general, if you're feeling depressed, the guesses are usually negative or upsetting. If you're feeling euphoric, your guesses are likely to be overly positive. If you're irritable, your guesses will stir up your anger. The conclusions you jump to usually match your mood. If you're anxious, you'll predict scary things. If you're jealous, you'll see betrayal even when it's not there. If you're angry, you'll assume that others have negative intentions.

The problem with jumping to conclusions is that they are often incorrect. When you act on them, you may be making a mistake. There are many different ways in which we jump to conclusions. These include mind reading, fortune-telling, catastrophizing, and personalization. As each is described, think of times when you may have thought the same way and later found out you were wrong.

In the pages that follow, you'll read descriptions of each of these ways that it is easy to jump to conclusions. Some of them might be familiar to you. Strategies are provided for correcting each thinking error before it causes you to overreact. As you read along, try to recall times when you might have jumped to conclusions in response to a stressful situation. The goal is for you to become more aware of when thinking errors are occurring so that you can intervene before you overreact. If you make it a habit to practice these methods, you'll find over time you will be less likely to jump to conclusions and, when they do occur, you'll be able to correct or dismiss these thoughts quickly.

Mind Reading

It's called *mind reading* when you try to guess what other people are thinking or feeling without asking them directly. This is a very common error in logic. The reason it is a thinking error is that the guesses are often based on emotion rather than on facts. You might look at a person and jump to conclusions based on how the person looks or dresses. The person might remind you of someone else in your life who looks or acts similarly so you assume this individual has the same thoughts and feelings. Or if you have known someone for a long time, you can get into the habit of assuming you know his or her thoughts.

Occasionally you will be correct. That's what gives you confidence that your "intuition" can be trusted. However, mind reading is a thinking error that can get you into trouble when it governs your actions and you turn out to be wrong. Here are some common examples. Do any of these sound like you?

> *Manic Mike:* "I know she's interested in me. She probably wore that dress just to get my attention."
> *Nervous Nellie:* "I don't need to ask. I can tell he's mad at me."
> *Depressed Doris:* "They probably think it's my fault that things didn't work out."
> *Hypomanic Hillary:* "They are just jealous because the teacher likes me best."

Try to jot down some of your own examples of mind reading in Exercise 7.2 below. Just think of a time you made a guess about someone and you turned out to be wrong. This might be a little difficult if you are convinced that you are right and not just jumping to conclusions. If you can't think of any examples, make it a point to pay attention to new thoughts you might have about other people. Pick someone you see regularly. Next time you see or talk to that person, try to monitor the guesses you are making about what he or she is thinking. Keep in mind that even the most talented psychotherapists can't read minds. They gather a lot of information about a person before they draw conclusions about them.

When you jump to conclusions, you're making guesses or assumptions about a situation, a problem, or a person. You might be convinced that your assumption is correct, but if emotion is influencing your thinking, you could be wrong. One of the biggest problems associated with mind reading is that it can cause arguments when you share your guesses and they sound more like accusations. Some examples that add fuel to an argument are:

EXERCISE 7.2 Mind Reading

In the space below, write down a few examples of when you might have made assumptions about what another person was thinking.

My own examples of mind reading:

- "I know what you're thinking."
- "You know I'm right."
- "I know you better than you know yourself."
- "I can tell you're mad."
- "You think you're smarter than everyone else."
- "You think you're perfect."

No matter whom you're talking to, mind reading can lead to bad feelings or start a fight. **The way to avoid mind reading and the conflict it can cause is to ask questions instead of making mind-reading statements.** When you're not upset, you probably do this automatically. When you're filled with strong emotions or when situations stimulate strong reactions in you, you may need to pause long enough to think things through more logically before you draw an accurate conclusion.

Think about the last time someone tried to read your mind and then incorrectly told you how you felt rather than asking you. It probably made you angry. Worse yet is jumping to conclusions and then acting on your assumptions without saying a word. Without open discussion, it is difficult to resolve differences.

Instead of mind reading, try asking questions such as the following:

- "What are you thinking?"
- "Do you agree with me?"
- "Because I know you pretty well, I would bet that you are feeling _____. Am I right?
- "Are you mad?"
- "I sometimes get the impression that you think you're smarter than me, and that really bothers me."
- "You may not realize this, but when you criticize me it's as if you're saying that you're perfect and I'm messed up. Is that what you think?"

Personalization

Personalization is jumping to the conclusion that a comment or situation has something to do with you when there are no facts to support this assumption. Depression can make you sensitive to criticism, especially if you are not feeling very good about yourself. This sensitivity can cause you to hear criticism from others even when it's not really there. People can jump to conclusions by taking things personally even when no blame is given. Personalization can make a person feel like the spotlight is on him or her. It is not as severe as paranoia, but it can be just as distressing. Here are some typical examples of personalization. Add some examples of your own to Exercise 7.3 on the next page.

Sensitive Sally: "My husband made that huffing sound before he asked me to pass the salt. I know him. That means he is disappointed with my cooking. I never seem to get it right."

EXERCISE 7.3 Personalization

In the space below, give some examples of times when you might have taken something personally without having all the facts.

My own examples of personalization:

Discouraged Denise: "It's my fault my son is in so much trouble at school. If only I had been a better mother."

Hyper Harvey: "Did you see how they looked at me when we walked in? They stopped talking for a second just to see what I would do next."

If you know that you have a tendency to take things personally when depressed or irritable, take that fact into consideration before you overreact. Here is an example of what Amanda has learned to say to herself to help her cope when it seems like she is being ignored at work.

"It feels like she ignored me on purpose, but I know that I'm kind of sensitive about that. Maybe she didn't see me, or maybe she had something else on her mind."

By taking your sensitivity into consideration, you open your mind to other explanations for events that are less personal than you originally thought. If you can consider all possibilities, you're in a better position to figure out the conclusion that is most likely to be true. If you have considered alternative explanations for your experience and you're still uncertain whether or not to take something personally, ask someone else's opinion or ask the person who upset you. Be sure the topic is worth discussing. Exercise 7.4 on the facing page includes a list of questions to consider when you catch yourself taking things personally. They can help you sort out what is real from what you imagine.

When Tommy overreacted to his mother's question about taking his medicine, his girlfriend helped him pose these questions to himself. His answers are on the next page.

Fortune-Telling

Fortune-telling is making predictions about future events. When your mood is down, you make negative predictions. These predictions seem realistic to you because your depression is

EXERCISE 7.4	Questions to Help Avoid Taking Things Personally

- Is it really about me?

- Could there be another explanation?

- Is it possible that it has nothing to do with me?

- Is it about the other person?

- Is it important enough to worry about?

- Is it important enough to discuss?

- Am I just being overly sensitive because I'm not doing so well right now?

making you feel negative. Therefore, the notion that something bad will happen is very easy to accept even when it is just a guess. Catastrophizing is an extreme version of fortune-telling where you jump to the conclusion that the worst possible outcome is bound to happen. Catastrophizing is fueled by anxiety and worry. Allowing yourself to believe that a catastrophe will occur usually makes your anxiety worse. When you're in this state, you panic and feel helpless to change the course of events. Not everyone catastrophizes when worried, but those

TOMMY'S EXAMPLE	Questions to Help Avoid Taking Things Personally

- **Is it really about me?** *Yes. It's about me and my medication.*

- **Could there be another explanation?** *Maybe I was looking wigged out. Maybe my mom was just worried about me.*

- **Is it possible that it has nothing to do with me?** *No, it was about me and my medicine, not anyone else's problem.*

- **Is it about the other person?** *My mom can't stay out of my life. She treats me like her baby still. She doesn't trust me to take care of myself. She has always been like that.*

- **Is it important enough to worry about?** *Probably not.*

- **Is it important enough to discuss?** *Maybe. I've told her to leave me alone about the medicine, but she doesn't listen to me. I can't talk to her on my own. Maybe I can get my dad to talk to her.*

- **Am I just being overly sensitive because I'm not doing so well right now?** *Possibly. I did kind of yell at her and storm out of there. I didn't used to be like that. I used to be able to deal with her better.*

who do tend to find that it's a common occurrence for them. Here are a few examples of negative fortune-telling. Add your examples to Exercise 7.5 at the bottom of the page.

Down-Hearted Donald: "It's not going to work out. Nothing works out for me."
Anxious Annie: "I'm going to make a fool of myself. I'll probably forget what I'm supposed to say and stand there staring at them like an idiot."
Worst-Case Wilber: "I made a huge mistake at work. I'm going to lose my job and not be able to pay my rent. I will be out on the street. No one hires a street person for a serious job. It's over for me."

Fortune-telling can also occur when your mood is elevated or euphoric; in this case the predictions are overly positive. Hypomania and mania can make you more self-confident than usual. You see opportunities but find it hard to see risks. You might jump to the conclusion that you can function well at work with little sleep, your new idea will make you bundles of money, or you should marry a person you've known for only a few weeks. In general, positive fortune-telling that is fueled by euphoria can lead to poor decision making. The impact may not be fully felt until the upward mood swing has passed and the rose-colored glasses of mania are no longer an influence. Think about how the following positive predictions might have negative consequences.

Hypomanic Harriet: "Once she hears this idea for making the office more efficient, I know she'll give me a raise, maybe even a promotion. I should be in charge. So what if I'm new on the job?"
Overconfident Oscar: "I just know I can ace that test without even having to open a book."
Euphoric Freddie: "She's the one I've waited for all my life. I don't care what Mom says. Two weeks with the girl of my dreams is long enough. We're getting married now."

To avoid fortune-telling errors, it's helpful to remember that just because your guess about what will happen next stirs up a lot of emotion does not mean that it's accurate. A

EXERCISE 7.5 **Fortune-Telling and Catastrophizing**

My own examples of fortune-telling and catastrophizing:

lot of people think their first thoughts reflect their instincts about a situation. If you think your instincts can be trusted when you're upset, you will latch on to the first ideas that come to mind. However, just because it was the first thing you thought of does not mean that it's right. In fact, your first thoughts in reaction to a stressful event are usually full of emotion, and emotions can distort your thinking. If you jump to the conclusion that something bad is going to happen and act on this first impression, you could easily be going down the wrong path. The solution to fortune-telling is to consider other possible outcomes rather than stop at your first guess.

Raquel and her boss have had a rocky relationship for many years. She admits to being overly sensitive when it comes to dealing with him. But there have been times in the past when he has taken advantage of her willingness to work hard or tried to cheat her on her salary or vacation pay. When she has to interact with him, she can't help feeling a little defensive. Feeling defensive can sometimes make her jump to conclusions about what he tells her. For example, he called her into his office to tell her that sales have been down this month and some changes would have to be made. She immediately thought, "We're not going to get the raises we were promised or the overtime pay. This company does not care about its employees. It only cares about the bottom line. I should just quit." Before she said anything, her boss went on to explain that they were going to change their product line and make fewer of the low-profit items and more of the higher-profit items. That would mean that Raquel needed to make some changes to the orders she had placed earlier that week.

Even though Raquel heard the instructions, she kept waiting for the other shoe to drop. She had not yet considered the possibility that she had jumped to conclusions. She was sure that bad news was coming. She left her boss's office but did not lower her guard. She stayed tense for weeks as they worked through the production changes, waiting for her boss to deliver the bad news. As it turned out, Raquel was wrong, and she had spent several stressful weeks waiting for her initial incorrect predictions to come to pass.

When you can catch yourself jumping to conclusions in response to a stressful situation, consider the other possible outcomes that could occur rather than stopping at the first one that comes to mind. Raquel, for example, could have also considered the possibility that her boss was telling the truth or that she was only partially right about the consequences. When you are uncertain about what will happen next in a stressful situation, try to get more information. Raquel could have saved herself a lot of worry if she had asked the boss directly about the raises and overtime pay. If he had bad news, as Raquel imagined, instead of spending several weeks worrying, she could have used the time to find a better solution or a way to cope with her circumstances.

Catastrophizing

Amanda has a tendency to catastrophize when stressed out. This year it was her turn to have her husband's family at the house for Christmas. She and her husband had managed to avoid this in the past because their house was too small. But now that they had a new and larger home, it was assumed that the whole family, including aunts, uncles, and cousins, would meet at Amanda's house for Christmas. Amanda does not have a good relationship with her in-laws. Her mother-in-law has always been very picky about food and was easily offended if Amanda and her husband did not buy her the right gift. The mother-in-law had been known to be judgmental and a gossip. Because of this, Amanda and her husband had decided to keep Amanda's illness a secret. Amanda was afraid that her mother-in-law would somehow find out that she had bipolar disorder when she visited for Christmas and would confront her in front of the whole family. Amanda convinced herself that her only hope was to put together such a perfect celebration that there would be no need to be nervous and no reason to question her sanity.

To reduce catastrophic thinking you have to get the situation into perspective and plan ahead for whatever happens. Getting something into perspective means seeing it for what it is, not magnifying, not jumping to conclusions, and not making inaccurate assumptions. If you know which outcome is most likely to occur, you can plan ahead for it. If you control the outcome, it may not turn out as bad as you think, or at least if you know with certainty that a situation is not going to turn out well, you can plan ahead to deal with the consequences. To control catastrophizing, work through the sequence of steps in Exercise 7.6 on the facing page. You may download and print additional copies of this exercise from *www.guilford.com/basco2-forms* and add them to your workbook as needed.

What's Next?

There were a lot of examples in this chapter of how the thoughts that come into your mind can strongly affect your mood. Catching these thoughts gives you an opportunity to think before you react. Rather than feeling like you have no control over your thoughts and actions, you can learn to slow the process, think through situations, and draw more logical and less emotional conclusions. The bottom line is that by learning to have more control over your thoughts and emotions, you can have more control over your actions. The reverse is true as well. In the next chapter you will begin to learn how changing your actions can help improve your mood and attitude. Not all of the exercises in this workbook will work every time. But if you have several tools—those that help you change your mood, thoughts, or actions—you will be better equipped to manage your symptoms.

How to Decatastrophize Your Thoughts

Follow the steps below to decatastrophize your scary thoughts.

1. If you think it's possible that you're catastrophizing about something, write down what you imagine will happen. It helps if you can picture the situation in your mind.

2. Ask yourself how likely it is that the catastrophe you imagined will occur. Is it a 100% certainty? Is there a 50% chance? Pick a number based on what you know to be true, not just what you fear.

    It is _____ % likely that the catastrophe I fear will actually happen.

3. Are there other outcomes, besides the one you imagined, that might be just as likely to occur? If so, what are the other possible options? Make a list.

    a.

    b.

    c.

    d.

    e.

    f.

4. Cross off the list the possibilities that are the least likely to occur. This might include your original fear.

5. Of the items remaining, choose the mostly likely outcome.

    The most likely outcome of this situation is _____

    _____

    _____

6. Is there anything you can do to make things turn out better? Is there anything others can do for you that would make the situation turn out better? If so, what are the possibilities?

7. If you are right and the situation turns out to be catastrophic, how will you cope? How can you prepare yourself to deal with the aftermath?

1. If you think it's possible that you're catastrophizing about something, write down what you imagine will happen. It helps if you can picture the situation in your mind.

   My mother-in-law will find out that I have bipolar disorder while she is visiting us, either by seeing my medication or because I am so uptight that I start acting hyper. My husband might also give it away. She will get upset about it and confront me in front of others. I will probably cry and not be able to handle it. I will be humiliated, and everyone else will be so uncomfortable that they'll leave early.

2. Ask yourself how likely it is that the catastrophe you imagined will occur. Is it a 100% certainty? Is there a 50% chance? Pick a number based on what you know to be true, not just what you fear.

   It is ___30___ % likely that the catastrophe I fear will actually happen.

3. Are there other outcomes, besides the one you imagined, that might be just as likely to occur? If so, what are the other possible options? Make a list.

   a. *She will be too caught up in the celebration to notice.*

   b. *If she does notice, she won't say anything.*

   c. *The event will go smoothly. I won't get nervous or hyper.*

   d. *I will get hyper, but she'll think it's normal for me.*

   e. *She already suspects that I have bipolar disorder and will say nothing.*

   f. *My husband will deal with her before she says anything to the other relatives.*

4. Cross off the list the possibilities that are least likely to occur, including your original fear.

   a. ~~*She will be too caught up in the celebration to notice.*~~

   b. *If she does notice, she won't say anything.*

   c. *The event will go smoothly. I won't get nervous or hyper.*

   d. ~~*I will get hyper, but she'll think it's normal for me.*~~

   e. ~~*She already suspects that I have bipolar disorder and will say nothing.*~~

   f. *My husband will deal with her before she says anything to the other relatives.*

5. Of the items remaining, choose the mostly likely outcome.

    The most likely outcome of this situation is   I will be nervous, but not hyper.

       If she thinks something is wrong, she will ask my husband and he

       will handle it for me.

6. Is there anything you can do to make things turn out better? Is there anything others can do for you that would make the situation turn out better? If so, what are the possibilities?

    If I'm prepared before everyone arrives, it will go better.

    I can make sure there is time for a short rest before everyone arrives, rather than scrambling until the last minute.

    I can take a Xanax if I feel that my anxiety is getting out of control.

    I can ask my husband to run interference with his mother if it looks like she is putting me on the spot.

7. If you are right and the situation turns out to be catastrophic, how will you cope? How can you prepare yourself to deal with the aftermath?

    If my mother-in-law starts to confront me, my husband will stop her. If he can't stop her, I will try to stay calm and address her concerns with a brief answer. I will offer to talk to her about my problems after the holiday is over. I'm sure she would agree to that. I will talk to my husband ahead of time about what to tell her and what not to tell her. I will schedule an appointment with my therapist for after Christmas just in case things do not go well.

8

Stop Avoidance
and Procrastination

In this chapter you will:

✓ Discover why you procrastinate.

✓ Learn to overcome your low motivation.

✓ Find out how to stop avoiding difficult tasks.

We all procrastinate, avoid, delay, or put off things at least some of the time. When it is a conscious act, sometimes it is for a logical reason like avoiding going outside because the weather is bad or putting off paying a bill because you know the check will bounce. In Chapter 4 you learned that people are not always aware of their feelings, so it is not uncommon to procrastinate or avoid things without knowing why. For example, perhaps you keep forgetting to make an appointment with the dentist or your gynecologist. You may not be consciously aware that you are avoiding it because it makes you feel anxious. In fact, if someone asked you if you were stalling, you might say that you are not avoiding the dentist or the doctor—you just have other things on your mind.

Procrastination and avoidance can cause big problems for people with bipolar disorder, especially if the things that are avoided are important or could make you feel better. This chapter will describe common reasons that people avoid and procrastinate and what you can do about it.

Inertia

- "I don't have the energy."
- "It's not worth it."
- "I can't get started."
- "I can't handle it."

Have any of these thoughts made you procrastinate when you were feeling depressed? Procrastination is very common when people are depressed. Feeling low usually includes having low energy. You can get fatigued easily and lose interest in your usual activities. This can cause you to avoid them or delay getting started. Unfortunately, doing less makes you feel worse about yourself or about life. This feeds your depression. The diagram at the bottom of the page shows you how this cycle can keep itself going.

To overcome procrastination, you have to find a way to break the cycle. This can be difficult if you've been stuck in this cycle for some time because of depression. You will probably take action only if you have a really good reason to do so. Take a minute and think of reasons it would be good for you to break your cycle of lethargy and inertia. Write down your reasons to take action in Exercise 8.1 on the next page. Amanda's reasons are that she has to take care of her children, she is tired of being in a funk, and she feels better about herself when she does something other than lie on the couch. Paul's reasons for getting out of a slump of inactivity are that he has a lot to do, things will only get worse the longer he neglects them, and he hates being different from everyone else. Raquel rarely gets into slumps anymore since she has learned to control her symptoms, but she disliked being lethargic in the past because even though she may have looked like she was resting, her guilt and self-criticism made it anything but restful.

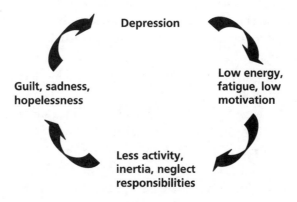

The cycle of lethargy and inertia.

EXERCISE 8.1 Reasons to Take Action
My Reasons to Take Action:

How to Get Moving

If you want to overcome avoidance or procrastination, you should start small and build up over time. The worst thing you can do is to try to go from always procrastinating to never procrastinating. It is too much to expect from yourself, and it runs a great risk of leading to failure. Hypomania and mania will make you think that you can and have to change everything about yourself at once. Don't let yourself be seduced by this idea.

Every activity starts with a small step. If you are avoiding something that causes you stress, the first step is to figure out what is causing your anxiety. It is possible that you are allowing your emotions to fuel scary thoughts like the thinking errors described in the last chapter. If you are avoiding an activity because you are afraid of the outcome, go back to Chapter 7 and work through the exercises for jumping to conclusions. When you are ready to take action, come back to this chapter and work through the exercises that follow.

If you are satisfied that anxiety is not the problem, perhaps you just need help to get yourself started. Overcoming procrastination starts with identifying a specific goal. If you did have the energy and the activity was worth it to you, what would you like to do? It doesn't really matter where you start; what matters is taking a step forward to break the cycle. Exercise 8.2 on the facing page provides you with some tips for taking action when procrastination has been holding you back.

Maria needs to lose some weight. She has put on a lot since she started taking medications for her mood swings, and she knows that diabetes and high blood pressure run in her family. Maria has been avoiding diets because just thinking about the restrictions makes her hungry. She has no faith that she can follow a diet, but she also knows that she has to stop avoiding the issue of her weight. Using the steps in Exercise 8.2, Maria decided to start small by adding exercise. The activity she chose was walking before she went to work in the morning. She set the goal of starting at the beginning of the next workweek. The cues she chose were to put her walking shoes, T-shirt, and sweatpants in her bathroom, where she would

EXERCISE 8.2	Tips for Getting Started

Follow the steps below to begin to break your cycle of lethargy and inertia to overcome avoidance and procrastination:

1. Start small.

2. Pick one activity at a time.

3. Decide when you will start.

4. Create cues to get started.

5. Review your list of reasons to take action (Exercise 8.1).

6. Ignore negative self-talk and take action even if you are not in the mood.

be sure to see them first thing in the morning. She wrote one reason to take action on an index card: her weight. Her negative self-talk about taking action started with "I don't want to." She made a note to herself to change the thought to "I don't want to, but I am going to do it anyway."

Activity Scheduling

There is something comforting about having a daily routine. You know what to expect. You do what you are supposed to do each day, and that can feel good. That's why some people find it helpful to get themselves on a schedule when they have fallen into a pattern of avoidance and procrastination. If you don't have a regular schedule of activities, such as work or school, it's easy to put things off. One of the major problems with avoidance and procrastination is that you might be missing out on things that would make you feel better about yourself or give you a sense of accomplishment. You also might be missing out on opportunities to have fun. Engaging in enjoyable activities can lift your mood. When that happens, you will often feel more energetic and motivated to take care of other aspects of your life. The same is true for things that give you a sense of accomplishment. Taking care of tasks that have been on your mind for a while will boost your self-confidence and make you feel better about yourself.

Exercise 8.3 comes in two parts (A and B) to give you enough space to complete it: an activity schedule for Sunday through Tuesday (p. 108) and one for Wednesday through Saturday (p. 109). You can make a schedule for the whole week or make plans one day at a time. To make the best use of activity schedules, make time the night before to plan for the following day. When you know what you'll be doing tomorrow, you avoid wasting time and prevent your low motivation from taking complete control. Some tips for completing your activity schedule are listed in Exercise 8.4 (at the top of p. 110). You may download and print additional copies of the schedules from *www.guilford.com/basco2-forms.*

Activity Schedule, Sunday–Tuesday

Put an X in the box after completing each task.

Time	Sun	Mon	Tues
9:00 A.M.	☐	☐	☐
10:00 A.M.	☐	☐	☐
11:00 A.M.	☐	☐	☐
12:00 P.M.	☐	☐	☐
1:00 P.M.	☐	☐	☐
2:00 P.M.	☐	☐	☐
3:00 P.M.	☐	☐	☐
4:00 P.M.	☐	☐	☐
5:00 P.M.	☐	☐	☐
6:00 P.M.	☐	☐	☐
7:00 P.M.	☐	☐	☐
8:00 P.M.	☐	☐	☐
9:00 P.M.	☐	☐	☐

Activity Schedule, Wednesday–Saturday

Put an X in the box after completing each task.

Time	Wed	Thur	Fri	Sat
9:00 A.M.	☐	☐	☐	☐
10:00 A.M.	☐	☐	☐	☐
11:00 A.M.	☐	☐	☐	☐
12:00 P.M.	☐	☐	☐	☐
1:00 P.M.	☐	☐	☐	☐
2:00 P.M.	☐	☐	☐	☐
3:00 P.M.	☐	☐	☐	☐
4:00 P.M.	☐	☐	☐	☐
5:00 P.M.	☐	☐	☐	☐
6:00 P.M.	☐	☐	☐	☐
7:00 P.M.	☐	☐	☐	☐
8:00 P.M.	☐	☐	☐	☐
9:00 P.M.	☐	☐	☐	☐

> **EXERCISE 8.4** **Tips for Completing Your Activity Schedule**
>
> - Fill in the time you plan to wake up and go to bed each day.
>
> - Write in regularly scheduled activities like work or appointments.
>
> - Plan at least one small pleasurable activity each day.
>
> - Schedule time to accomplish one task each day.
>
> - Be realistic with your planning. Don't schedule too much.

People

- "I don't want people to see me."
- "I don't want to hear what they have to say."
- "I can't deal with people right now."
- "They can't tell me what to do."

Do you avoid people? Do any of the reasons above sound familiar? When you get depressed, you may not feel like being around others. It may seem like too much hassle, people might seem annoying or uncaring, or you might not want them to know what's going on with you. Perhaps you feel anxious about how you'll act or how others will treat you. Although avoiding social situations is a natural urge, it is probably one of the worst things you can do when depressed. Isolation breeds loneliness. Loneliness fuels depression. Depression makes you want to isolate yourself even more. It can become a vicious cycle, as shown in the diagram below. While you are alone you have too much time to dwell on your misery, you have no one to talk you out of your negative thinking, and you miss opportunities to laugh. In spite of the fact that family members or friends do not always say the right things, you need them for support or at least for a distraction from your emotional pain.

The solution is to do the opposite of what you feel like doing. Instead of avoiding people move toward them. Let people know you're feeling down. Call on a friend, a family member, someone from your place of worship, a support group member, a coworker, your therapist or doctor, or a neighbor. Don't hide. Let people reach out to you and offer their aid. They may not be able to solve your problems, but they can stand by your side to give you the added strength you might need to solve your own problems.

This is easier said than done. To stop avoiding people you may need to psych yourself up. Use Exercise 8.5 on the facing page to think of several reasons why it would be good for

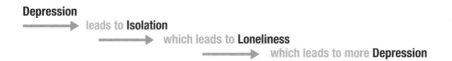

EXERCISE 8.5   Good Reasons to Interact with People

When I have contact with people, I get these positives out of it:

PAUL'S EXAMPLE   Good Reasons to Interact with People

When I have contact with people, I get these positives out of it:

I temporarily forget about my problems.

They can make me laugh.

I can get out of myself for a little while.

Afterward I'm always glad I did it.

AMANDA'S EXAMPLE   Good Reasons to Interact with People

When I have contact with people, I get these positives out of it:

They remind me that I do have support if I want it.

I get a reality check from my overly negative thinking. My family tells me I'm not as worthless as I think and I'm not alone in my misery.

Going to church with others gives me hope.

you to spend time with other people. Think of times in the past when socializing was good for you. Try to pinpoint what you enjoyed about it, how it improved your mood, or other ways that the people in your life helped you cope with your mood swings.

Uncertainty

- "I don't know what to do."
- "I don't know where to start."
- "I might make the wrong decision."
- "I don't know if it's worth it."

As a nurse, Amanda is very organized at work, follows a routine, and expects everyone she supervises to do the same. She is a perfectionist when she is feeling fine, but her all-or-nothing approach crumbles when she is going through periods of severe depression. When she can't do it all, she tends to do nothing. She procrastinates at home, avoids people except for her immediate family, and allows tasks and responsibilities to pile up. She knows that her problems will not go away, chores will not disappear, and bills will not magically get paid, but she feels powerless to take action. She completely loses her direction.

When Amanda has lost a job because of depression, job hunting feels overwhelming. She is not sure whether she is better off waiting until she feels better to start looking for a job or starting right away. She wonders whether she should stay in nursing or try something easier. She's afraid of making the wrong choice, so she thinks about giving up and going on disability. Uncertainty keeps her stuck.

Depression makes normal everyday activities and decisions feel overwhelming. In these circumstances the natural tendency for many people is to procrastinate, delay, or avoid action. Procrastination is one of the short-term coping behaviors that was described in Chapter 5. It may relieve your stress in the short run but can make things more complicated or difficult in the long run. The problem is finding your way out of procrastination when your symptoms of depression are interfering with your concentration, energy, decision-making ability, and self-confidence. Until your symptoms have improved, you have to rely on strategies that work around the feeling of being overwhelmed, like those in Exercise 8.6 on the facing page. This can help you avoid procrastination. You may download and print additional copies of the lists from *www.guilford.com/basco2-forms*.

"A" List and "B" List

When you are feeling so overwhelmed with life that it is easier to avoid everything than to take action, you need a way to make your responsibilities feel less burdensome. Exercise 8.6 will help you reduce your long to-do list to something shorter and easier to accomplish. The goal is to make two short lists each day: (1) things you absolutely have to do and (2) things you would like to do if you have the time and energy. The things you must do become your

EXERCISE 8.6 "A" List and "B" List
In the spaces below, make a list of no more than three things you would like to accomplish today. Choose things that are easy to complete or list small steps toward a larger goal.

My "A" List

Things I need to do today

1.

2.

3.

On your "B" list, add no more than three things that you would like to do after you finish your "A" list tasks. These can be chores or pleasurable activities.

My "B" List

Things I'd like to do when I finish my "A" list

1.

2.

3.

From *The Bipolar Workbook, Second Edition.* Copyright 2015 by The Guilford Press.

"A" list. You should never have more than a few items on that list for any day. "A" list items are things that cannot wait, such as paying a bill, getting food from the store, or attending an appointment. "A" list items can also include mental activities such as making time to think, plan, or figure out how to solve a problem.

The items on your "B" list will include things you would like to do if you have enough time and energy. They do not absolutely have to be done that day, but if time and energy permit, you would really like to do them. This might include running an errand ahead of time rather than waiting until it's urgent or refilling a prescription before you take the last pill. "B" list items can also be fun activities like visiting a friend, working on a hobby, or reading a book for enjoyment. There should never be more than a few items on your "B" list for any one day, especially if your "A" list is likely to take a lot of time.

AMANDA'S EXAMPLE   "A" List and "B" List
My "A" List
Things I need to do today
1. Make the kids' lunches before I go to sleep
2. Shower and put on clean clothes
3. Put the dishes in the dishwasher
My "B" List
Things I'd like to do when I finish my "A" list
1. Wash one load of laundry—underwear
2. Call the windshield repair company to schedule a repair on my car
3. Look online for nursing jobs

The goal is to try to finish your "A" list activities before you begin your "B" list activities. This will allow you to do the most important things first, solve critical problems, and have a sense of accomplishment. Any leftover items can be carried over to the next day.

People like Amanda have to be careful not to put too many things on either list. Amanda has always been a list maker, but she usually has lists that are several pages long. When she is not depressed, she can do a lot. Lowering her standards temporarily to a few "A" list and "B" list items will be a challenge. She has to convince herself that it is OK to do less than usual until she feels better. That means giving up her "all or nothing" approach, at least for a while, and substituting a "little bit at a time" approach. The exercises in Chapters 7, 10, and 11 will help her with the self-critical thinking that may get in the way.

Fear

- "It is going to be stressful."
- "I don't know how to handle the situation."
- "I don't trust myself to do the right thing."
- "It's going to make me feel worse."

As you learned in Chapter 7, it is easy to scare yourself into avoidance. You learned how to work through the tendency to jump to conclusions. If you think you are avoiding things or procrastinating because you are afraid of a bad outcome, go back to Chapter 7, find the thinking error that fits your situation, and work through your scary thoughts before you make a plan to take action.

No one likes to deal with unpleasant situations, but emotions can color thinking in ways that make it seem like taking action would lead to catastrophe. You can test your fearful thoughts using the strategies in Chapter 7 as well as those coming up in Chapters 10 and 11. When you are ready to take action, try using the "A" list and "B" list method you learned in Exercise 8.6.

Pleasure

- **"I'd rather play than work."**
- **"I finally feel good and want to have fun."**
- **"I deserve a chance to relax and do nothing."**
- **"I don't want to lose the high."**

Miguel is a pleasure seeker even when he is not hypomanic. He has a fun-loving personality and would rather play than work. He puts a lot of effort into his job and pays his bills, so he thinks he deserves to play hard on his time off. His wife, Desiree, doesn't disagree in principle, but she also works full time and thinks they should share responsibility for household chores, yard work, car maintenance, and all the other little things that grown-ups have to do. When she reminds him to do his half of the chores, Miguel accuses her of sounding like his mother.

Miguel is almost 40, but he considers himself a kid at heart. He still abides by the philosophy that it is better to ask for forgiveness than permission, especially when it is his wife he is talking about. This means that he procrastinates on the "grown-up" things Desiree wants him to do and then asks forgiveness when he stays out all day fishing with his friends. When he is hypomanic, the day of fishing turns into a weekend outing with his buddies, often with too much alcohol.

Miguel has procrastinated and avoided chores in the past with no problem. He did so when he was still living with his parents, knowing that his mother would eventually do his chores for him because she couldn't stand the mess. She would get mad, and he would apologize and promise to do better next time. That is how the pattern started.

Now that he is married, Miguel's procrastination is a problem for his wife. Desiree hates to fight because her parents used to fight all the time. She doesn't want to be like them, so she avoids conflict and tries to forgive Miguel's behavior. She forgave him when he lost his job, when his drinking led to jail for a DUI, and when he has missed their anniversary and her birthday. Desiree's avoidance of confrontation is as much the problem as Miguel's procrastination with chores.

Find the Middle Ground

What Miguel and Desiree have in common is that they both want to avoid something negative. They are not too depressed or afraid to take action. They are not trying to avoid one another, and they are not uncertain about what to do. It is simply that neither of them wants to engage in an unpleasant activity. He doesn't want to do work at home on the weekends, and she doesn't want to fight about it. Unfortunately, avoidance is going to take a toll on their marriage.

Pleasure seekers get immediate positive feedback from doing pleasant things. It feels good. If you are someone who has periods of depression, you know what a relief it is to feel good. It is easy to understand why Miguel wants to make the most of every depression-free moment. Similarly, it is easy to understand why Desiree doesn't want to fight with Miguel. Arguments result in immediate negative feedback and are extremely unpleasant. Where they are stuck is that Miguel and Desiree are using an all-or-nothing approach. Miguel assumes that all chores will be unpleasant and should be avoided. Desiree assumes that any discussion about the chores will end in a fight like the ones her parents used to have. Coping with avoidance in both of their cases has to do with finding a middle ground, a compromise between the extremes of going all out and doing nothing at all.

Because it is not our problem, it is fairly easy to see what Miguel and Desiree need to do. They are reasonable people who care about one another. Both want to have a good life, including a good marriage. They need to talk about a compromise that allows them to each achieve their goals. Since Desiree is the one who is aware that there is a problem, she has responsibility for bringing it up. But to avoid a confrontation, she is dealing with it by avoiding all conversation about Miguel's behavior—that's her all-or-nothing approach.

One of the reasons people like Desiree feel stuck is that they believe they have to solve problems all by themselves—another all-or-nothing idea. They forget that there are others who can help. To find the middle ground with Miguel, Desiree needs advice on how to start the conversation and keep it from escalating into an all-out fight. She can ask family members or friends for advice, but they are not always going to be neutral. Miguel sees a psychiatrist for his medications. She is another resource.

Clinicians can make good referees. If Desiree wants to talk about Miguel's behavior in a safe environment with someone who will help keep them on track, she can ask to join Miguel at his next counseling session or doctor's visit. Below is an example of how Desiree made this happen.

DESIREE: Miguel, I want to go with you to your next visit with the psychiatrist.

MIGUEL: OK. Why do you want to go?

DESIREE: We need to talk about the chores, but I don't want to fight.

MIGUEL: Not that again.

DESIREE: I think we need some help to resolve this. I don't want to fight about it. I want to find a solution. We haven't been able to resolve it on our own. Let's ask for some help before it ruins our marriage. I love you, and I don't want to end up like my parents.

MIGUEL: Fine.

In Chapter 10 you will learn another approach to dealing with all-or-nothing ideas: addressing the logic behind these types of thoughts. If this is a common problem for you, read ahead to that chapter.

What's Next?

Procrastination and avoidance are both common coping behaviors. They help people deal with unpleasant things or situations, uncertainty, and fear. They are common reactions to the lethargy that comes with depression. Avoidance and procrastination can reduce stress in the short run but will not solve your problems in the long run. This chapter focused on helping you figure out what is causing you to procrastinate and offered strategies for breaking the cycle of lethargy and inertia. In the next chapter you will learn to deal with another problem that can keep you stuck— feeling too overwhelmed to take action.

Step 4

Reduce
Your Symptoms

9

Regain Control
When You Feel Overwhelmed

In this chapter you will:

✓ Learn how to cope with feeling overwhelmed.

✓ Find out how to control your environment by reducing overstimulation.

✓ Discover ways to improve your sleep.

Feeling Overwhelmed

The amount of stress you can handle will vary from day to day. When you have slept well, have energy, and are able to concentrate, it is easier to handle the multitude of tasks and responsibilities that you face. When you are tired, stressed, and have too many things to think about at one time, it is much harder to cope. When your ability to cope is limited and you have many things to do, it is common to feel overwhelmed. Being overwhelmed can feel like a combination of fatigue and sadness. Sometimes there is irritability and agitation as well as mental fuzziness. You might know exactly what to do but can't make yourself do it. And just thinking about the number of steps needed to accomplish a goal may leave you feeling exhausted and discouraged.

When people feel overwhelmed, they often procrastinate or avoid chores or tasks altogether, as described in the examples in Chapter 8. This usually results in getting further and further behind. Knowing that chores are stacking up can worsen your mood, especially if it makes you feel bad about yourself. Procrastinating or avoiding a task altogether usually reduces the bad feelings at least temporarily. That is why we do it. Here's how it works:

1. When you get overwhelmed, you tell yourself, "I can't handle it," and you feel extremely tense. When you walk away from something you need to do and tell yourself, "I'll do it later," you feel more relaxed.
2. When you do this, you are conditioning yourself to associate difficult tasks with feeling bad and walking away from them with feeling better. Because of this conditioning, the next time you are faced with a difficult problem you are more likely to walk away than to try to handle it. This is how you create a bad habit.
3. When you do this over and over again, you lose confidence in yourself and your ability to cope.
4. When your confidence is low, you are less likely to make yourself deal with stressful situations.
5. In the meantime, problems or tasks can get bigger, harder to handle, and more overwhelming.
6. All of this makes you feel worse.

The best way to handle this situation is to break it down and take it on!

How to Break It Down and Take It On

The way to cope with the feeling of being overwhelmed and still make some progress toward your goals is to change the way you look at a task or problem. Whether you're talking about cleaning a house you've neglected for months, catching up on your income tax filing, or getting a job, you can turn a big overwhelming task into smaller, more manageable parts. It's all in how you look at it.

If you see a messy apartment as a disaster area that will take weeks to clean, it can seem too overwhelming to take on. If you want to find a job but think about all the little things that must be done to prepare yourself to work, to find available positions, and to convince someone to hire you, the sheer magnitude of the task can stop you in your tracks. When you're depressed, if your motivation is low, you can't imagine how to begin. If your concentration is poor, you may not be able to keep your mind focused long enough to get organized. If your energy is low, you may be too tired to do the work. All of this taken together contributes to your feeling completely overwhelmed.

Feeling low or depressed + A big task to do = Feeling overwhelmed

If solving a big problem would make you feel better, then try the steps in the next section to break down your problem into smaller and more manageable parts and take it on one step at a time.

HOW TO BREAK IT DOWN

- **Step 1: Don't tell yourself that it has to be done all at once.** You might prefer to do the whole thing in one day, but this may not be reasonable. In Exercise 9.1 below, write out some reminders to yourself that might help you set realistic goals for getting things done.

Amanda is a bit of a perfectionist and expects herself to be on top of things at all times. When she has tried to tell herself that it was OK to do a small amount of work at a time, it didn't work because another part of her responded by saying that she *should* be able to get it all done. This is because she can do all her household chores in one day when she isn't depressed. If you are like Amanda, you may have to work at cutting yourself some slack. It's better to do a small amount of work than to do nothing at all. Something is better than nothing. Try saying that to yourself when your perfectionism makes you set unreasonable expectations.

- **Step 2: Write down all the major steps involved** in solving your problem or completing your task. You may not like writing things down, but taking it out of your head and putting it on paper will help you feel less overwhelmed. Try writing down your ideas in Exercise 9.2 on the next page and see if it works for you.

Tommy found it helpful to write out a list of steps it would take to get caught up with a research paper he needed to write for class. When he broke it down, it seemed more manageable to him. Amanda, on the other hand, started to write down the steps it would take to clean her house and got overwhelmed by the number of things she had to do. She put down the list and just started cleaning the house. It worked better for her to go on to Step 3.

- **Step 3: Pick a place to start.** There may be an obvious first step, but in most cases doing anything, even if it is out of sequence, is better than doing nothing. If you feel the urge to do more than one step, try to resist it. If you take on too much, you will feel overwhelmed

---

EXERCISE 9.1 Self-Talk to Do One Thing at a Time

Things I can say to myself about doing one thing at a time:

(e.g., *Even if I can't do it all, doing something is better than doing nothing.*)

EXERCISE 9.2   Things You Want to Accomplish
The steps I want to accomplish:

all over again. Pick your first step and write it down in Exercise 9.3 at the bottom of the page. Seeing it in writing can help you keep your commitment to yourself.

Raquel gets behind on paying bills from time to time. She hates the task because it always reminds her of what little money she has. Because she has had a long-standing habit of avoiding paying bills, she does not have an organized system for keeping the bills together, knowing where her checkbook is, or knowing the due dates of each payment. In the past, she thought about trying to create a system, but that would take more time than she wanted to spend on it. Although an organized system might be a good idea, it is not where she wanted to start. Instead, Raquel decided that her first steps would be to find her checkbook and her bills. Throughout the day, as she found a bill she stopped and wrote a check for it and put it in an envelope to mail. Raquel knew it was not the most efficient way to go about it, but at least it got done.

HOW TO TAKE IT ON

• **Step 1: Pick a day and time to start.** Make an appointment with yourself to begin the first step of your chore. Choose a time that is realistic, when lots of interruptions are unlikely to occur and your other obligations are unlikely to interfere. Schedule it for when you are likely to have time and energy.

EXERCISE 9.3   Pick a Place to Start
This is where I am going to start:

• **Step 2: Do the first step** even if you're not in the mood, not feeling motivated, or can think of a dozen other things you would rather do. Tell yourself that making a little bit of progress is better than making no progress at all.

Many people complain about being unmotivated and uninterested in taking care of unpleasant tasks, especially when just thinking about it makes them feel overwhelmed. They put things off until they feel motivated to act, but that feeling rarely comes. There is no real magic to increasing your motivation or making yourself take action. When it comes down to it, it's just a matter of deciding that it's in your best interest to take action. You take the first step despite all of your resistance and excuses because you believe it's the right thing to do. For that moment, you ignore the negative emotions that paralyze you and just get started. Once you see yourself act, your motivation will begin to return.

• **Step 3: Cross each step off the list as it is completed.** Give yourself a pat on the back or treat yourself to something fun or pleasurable for taking some action. Avoid telling yourself that it doesn't matter because you have so much more to do. You have to make the work worthwhile. If you are someone who is motivated by the relief you feel when something gets done, completing the task may be the only reward you need. If the task you are trying to do is difficult for you and does not give you a lot of pleasure, you will have to find another way to give yourself positive reinforcement for getting it done. This is an important step because it gives you a reason to go on with the next part of the task. Think of a possible reward to give to yourself. It does not have to be a huge or expensive reward. Allowing yourself a rest, eating an ice-cream cone, or watching your favorite TV show can be rewarding. Plan ahead for your reward and write it down in Exercise 9.4 below as a reminder.

- Raquel's reward for getting the bills paid was having a short nap.
- Amanda's reward for taking action toward her goals is getting a break from self-criticism for her procrastination.
- Tommy's reward for finishing the term paper will be taking the night off and going to a movie.

• **Step 4: Select the next part** of the task to do and schedule a time to do it. Repeat steps 1 through 4 until you are done. When you have completed your task, give yourself some credit and a reward, or brag to someone who will understand what you've accomplished!

EXERCISE 9.4 **Possible Rewards**

When I am able to take action, I will give myself the following reward:

Disqualifying the Accomplishment

Raquel thinks that feeling depressed is no excuse for not getting things done. She doesn't cut herself any slack for having low energy at times or difficulty concentrating. She breaks down tasks into smaller pieces when she gets overwhelmed and stuck, but when she accomplishes each piece, instead of giving herself praise, she criticizes herself for not having finished the task sooner or not having done a better job.

Beating yourself up for accomplishing tasks is not a way to stay motivated. If you were coaching someone else—for example, a child or a student—you would not berate the person for not completing the tasks sooner or better. If you did, the child or student would stop performing for you. You are no different.

Not allowing yourself to feel good about small accomplishments can do you more harm than good. When you struggle with mood swings and all the other symptoms of bipolar disorder, every accomplishment, even the small ones, can take great effort. If this sounds like you, try not to defeat yourself by expecting more than is reasonable. Sometimes you have to pat yourself on the back just for getting up in the morning because sometimes getting yourself out of bed *is* a major accomplishment.

How to Reduce Overstimulation

There are two sources of stimulation that can make mania and hypomania worse. The first group includes stimulation from your environment, such as noise (see the table below), and the second is internal stimulation that comes from having a lot of thoughts or ideas (see the table on p. 127). Too much external stimulation can make you feel overwhelmed. It can worsen racing thoughts and make it hard for you to concentrate. Overstimulation can keep you awake at night. Even positive things such as people laughing and having fun can be mentally overstimulating at times. Things in your environment that can overstimulate you are listed in the following table.

Sometimes your own thoughts and activities can be overstimulating. For example, if you're beginning to have symptoms of mania or hypomania, you might have more ideas than usual and you might be more creative as well. The more you think about your new ideas, the more stimulated you become. Emotions such as joy or excitement may seem to escalate the process, especially if you try to put your ideas into action. The more excited you get, the

Sources of Overstimulation in Your Environment			
Noise	Too many people	Loud music	Children playing
Clutter	Traffic on the road	Phones ringing	Group therapy
Confusion	Loud laughter	Babies crying	TV commercials

Examples of Internal Overstimulation	
Racing thoughts	Starting new projects
Rumination about problems or worries	Mulling over creative thoughts or ideas
Reminiscing about the past, especially emotional events	Repeating thoughts to store in memory instead of writing them down
Making plans for new activities or adventures	Rewinding bad events

faster your ideas will flow. This might actually feel good until you become overly stimulated, have more thoughts than you can handle, and begin to feel agitated or exhausted. Unfortunately, it's hard to stop the process when it has gone on too long.

People like Raquel's brother Stan, who hears voices during periods of mania and depression, find that this symptom is worse when there is a lot of noise or activity in their environments. In addition to taking medication, reducing overstimulation can help.

Reduce Environmental Stimulation

The first step in reducing overstimulation is to **recognize** that it is occurring. You might be aware of feeling uptight, anxious, or unsettled, but you might not always recognize its source. Amanda can feel herself tightening up when the kids are fighting. The second step is to **identify** the source of stimulation. Is it something in your environment or something within you? In Amanda's case it's her kids. The third step is to **take action**. Amanda can redirect the kids' activities so that they do something less noisy, or she can leave the room until she feels more able to handle it.

If the source of stimulation is something in your environment, find a way to quiet it down or distance yourself from it. This might mean lowering the volume on the television or radio, walking away from a crowd of people, or asking children to play more quietly. Find a quiet place to gather your thoughts and calm yourself. You can go to another room, take a quiet walk, turn out the lights and lie down, or sit in your car for a while.

If a cluttered environment is the source of overstimulation, you can leave it or you can try to fix it. To fix it, apply the step-by-step procedures under "How to Break It Down" and "How to Take It On" earlier in this chapter for gaining control over your environment by fixing one thing at a time.

Reduce Internal Stimulation

In many ways it's easier to control external stimulation than it is to control internal stimulation. You can walk away from a busy environment, but you can't easily walk away from a busy mind. To reduce internal stimulation you have to find a way to quiet your mind or organize your thoughts. The goal is to slow your mental processes so they are no longer overstimulating. Here are some ideas:

GET QUIET

Taking action to quiet your environment is a good first step. If there is less noise on the outside, there will be less confusion in your head. Follow the instructions in the previous section for reducing external stimulation.

CALM YOURSELF

Mental overstimulation seems to be fueled by strong emotions such as anxiety or excitement. Use a relaxation exercise to reduce tension in your body, distract yourself for a while with soothing music, or put your feet up and rest for a short while. Anything that has relaxed you or helped you wind down when you were stressed can usually reduce mental overstimulation. It is recommended, however, that you avoid alcohol as a solution.

GET ORGANIZED

One of the symptoms of hypomania and mania is having an increased number of ideas for new activities or adventures. Sometimes you feel a surge of motivation that makes you want to take care of neglected chores, begin a creative task, or make a change in some aspect of your life. It may seem like one new idea just leads to another. This can feel good, especially if you've been suffering from depression recently and your thoughts have been slow or your motivation has been low. But if you don't set a limit on internal stimulation, it can reach a point where you have too many ideas and your thoughts become disorganized and distressing. To control the urge to follow each new idea when it comes to mind, try Exercise 8.6, "A" List and "B" List on page 113.

Get a Good Night's Sleep

Another way to feel more in control is to get enough sleep. Exercise 9.5 on the facing page includes strategies you can use to ensure a good night's sleep. If you're doing all you can to sleep well and still have insomnia, talk to your doctor about sleep aids.

What If I Can't Fall Asleep?

Just as there are things you can do to help yourself get a good night's sleep, there are a number of things you probably should *not* do. Things that can interfere with a good night's sleep

EXERCISE 9.5 Steps for a Good Night's Sleep
If you are having difficulty falling asleep at night, try the following steps.
Be consistent: Try to go to bed and wake up at about the same time each day, even on weekends.
It's a nighttime thing: Avoid sleeping during the day and staying awake late at night. If your sleep cycle is already switched around, work with your doctor on a plan for getting your sleep back to normal.
Keep your bed a place for sleep: Make it a habit to watch TV, eat, read, or pay your bills in another room, at a table, or on a couch. Teach your body to associate going to bed with falling asleep.
Get comfortable: Make your sleep area comfortable by picking pillows, blankets, and clothing that make you feel good.
Gear down for the night: Start preparing to sleep at least an hour ahead of time by quieting your environment and quieting your mind.
Avoid stimulants that might keep you awake: A hot cup of cocoa or coffee, a few cigarettes, or some dessert might sound good at nighttime, but for those who are sensitive to caffeine, nicotine, or sugar, they may make it harder to fall asleep. If you have any digestive problems, late dinners or spicy meals might trouble your stomach and keep you awake.

are listed in Exercise 9.6 on the next page. Make a plan to avoid these things when you have trouble falling asleep.

DON'T PANIC

Anxiety and sleep are not a good mix. Starting to worry or even panic about your inability to sleep will only make it harder to fall asleep. Sleep happens automatically. It is not a thing you can easily will your body to do, so the harder you work at convincing yourself to fall asleep, the longer it can take. Not being able to fall asleep can also leave you frustrated and even aggravated. Strong emotions like this are not conducive to falling asleep.

CALM YOUR BODY

Your body and your mind work together to help you fall asleep. If your mind is too busy to settle down, you can help the process along by trying to relax your body. Start with your toes and work toward your head. Focus on letting go of tensions in each muscle and getting your body into a comfortable position. Work on one foot at a time, then one leg at a time, and so on. Make sure you relax the muscles in your face, especially your forehead, jaw, and eyes.

EXERCISE 9.6   Things *Not* to Do When You Are Having
Trouble Sleeping

Below is a list of common things that can interfere with your sleep and recommendations for coping with them. Try the ones that apply to you.

Caffeine: Don't make yourself a pot of coffee. The caffeine can keep you awake. If you enjoy a hot cup of coffee on a cold night, buy some decaffeinated coffee for evening and nighttime use.

Internet: Avoid getting out of bed to surf the Internet. Instead of getting sleepy, you will most likely stimulate your brain and keep yourself awake.

TV and books: If you are going to watch television or read a book, choose something that is not likely to keep you awake. A boring book or a television rerun will do the trick. Avoid shows with people arguing, cliffhangers, violence, or real-life docudramas.

Chores: Don't get up and clean your house. Although unfinished chores may be on your mind, the process of doing physical labor in the middle of the night will tense your muscles rather than relax them. To be mentally alert enough to do chores you have to stay awake. This defeats the purpose of getting a good night's sleep.

Exercise: It is probably not a good idea to get out of bed to exercise even if you know that exercise can wear you out. Physical activity can overstimulate your mind and body. If exercise is usually a good idea for you, schedule time before you go to bed to work out.

After you have relaxed from head to toe, count to ten slowly and with each number try to let go and relax just a little bit more. Search for any remaining tension and release it. If you like this kind of strategy, you may want to try the more elaborate relaxation exercise provided in Chapter 15.

TOO ALERT TO FALL ASLEEP

If you're too wide awake to fall asleep, you would be better off getting out of bed and doing something else relaxing, like watching television, reading a book, or any other activity that usually calms you or tires your mind.

Reduce Nighttime Worry and Rumination

As you begin to relax your body to fall asleep, sometimes your mind will wander over the events of the day, conversations with other people, or problems that you face. It seems involuntary. The thoughts just pop into your head, and one idea can lead to another. Pretty soon you can find yourself more mentally alert than before you went to bed. If you frequently have this kind of bedtime experience, it's time to try something new. Here are the steps to control nighttime worry and rumination.

- **Step 1: Make time to review your day**, your worries, and your problems before you go to bed, preferably more than an hour before bedtime. Raquel liked to set aside time before the evening news. Watching the news made it easier for her to let go of her day and get ready for bed.

- **Step 2: Make a list.** As you begin to think about the things that bother you, write them down. If you see them in writing, you won't need to keep them in your head. You can use any piece of paper to make the list, or you can use the space in Exercise 9.7 below to practice this exercise. You can also download and print additional copies of the Daily Review List from *www.guilford.com/basco2-forms*. Raquel's list is on the next page.

- **Step 3: Prioritize.** Try to put the items on your list in some sort of order according to their importance. Little things can sometimes feel like they have great importance because they happened most recently or because they were really annoying. Make the order of worries reflect the significance of items in the grand scheme of your life. On the bottom of page 132 is how Raquel prioritized her list.

EXERCISE 9.7 Daily Review List

In the space below, make a list of the issues, problems, people, or ideas that are on your mind. Use just enough words to help you remember the issue; don't write out the whole problem. The order is not important.

My Daily Review List

RAQUEL'S EXAMPLE Daily Review List

My Daily Review List

I got up too late.

The boss was in a bad mood.

The dog didn't eat all his food today.

My skirt felt too tight. I'm gaining weight again.

Call Mom this weekend and try to cheer her up.

Don't forget to return the DVDs.

Getting up on time, rated number 1, was important because it made the rest of her day go more smoothly. Raquel skipped numbers 2 through 4 and gave her second item a ranking of 5 to remind herself that the next item is not very important in the grand scheme of things. The other items were not all that important to Raquel and certainly were not worth losing sleep over.

- **Step 4: Make a plan of action** for the items that bother you the most. Think of something you can do tomorrow to take a step toward its solution even if it means you will only schedule time to think about it more, talk to someone about it, or get more information on the subject. You don't have to feel burdened with resolving big issues all at once. Think about a logical first step by considering your options and select one that might help you achieve your goals. Write down your plan so that you will not have to hold it in your memory. Raquel wrote down a few ideas for the items she thought she could control (see facing page).

RAQUEL'S EXAMPLE WITH PRIORITIES Daily Review List

My Daily Review List

(1) I got up too late.

(5) The boss was in a bad mood.

(3) The dog didn't eat all his food today.

(2) My skirt felt too tight. I'm gaining weight again.

(4) Call Mom this weekend and try to cheer her up.

(6) Don't forget to return the DVDs.

RAQUEL'S EXAMPLE WITH SOLUTIONS　　Daily Review List

My Daily Review List

(1) I got up too late. Set the alarm clock for 15 minutes earlier.

(5) The boss was in a bad mood. Nothing I can do.

(3) The dog didn't eat all his food today. Talk to kids about not giving him snacks.

(2) My skirt felt too tight. I need to stay away from bread for a while.

(4) Call Mom this weekend and try to cheer her up. I may not be able to make her feel better.

(6) Don't forget to return the DVDs. Put them in the car before you forget.

• **Step 5: Stop the thought.** If what you are ruminating about is not very important or is beyond your control, but keeps popping into your head, tell yourself to "Stop." Use a forceful tone with yourself, even if it's only in your thoughts. Remind yourself that rumination is a waste of your energy. Refocus your thoughts and energy on something worthwhile or within your realm of control. If that doesn't work, try switching your thought to something more pleasant, like remembering a walk in the park or the last time you saw a beautiful sunset.

What's Next?

During periods of depression, hypomania, and mania, it is common to feel overwhelmed. The causes can include overstimulation from noise or activity in your environment, too much mental activity, or more responsibilities than you have the energy to handle. Feeling overwhelmed can make you procrastinate or avoid things that are stressful and can interfere with your sleep. This chapter described several things that you can do to reduce stimulation, get a good night's sleep, and take on the tasks that are on your mind. In the next chapter you will learn more about how to improve your symptoms by changing your negative outlook. Changes in outlook can lead to positive changes in your actions.

10

Change Your Negative Outlook

In this chapter you will:

✓ Find out how to keep yourself from magnifying negative thoughts.

✓ Discover strategies for overcoming tunnel vision.

✓ Learn to overcome all-or-nothing thinking.

In Chapter 7 you learned about a very common type of thinking error called jumping to conclusions. This occurs when you make guesses about people, situations, or circumstances even when there are few facts to support your ideas—the type of guess depends on your mood. In other words, you fill in the blanks with bad guesses when in a bad mood and good guesses when in a good mood. Sometimes you get lucky and you are right, but incorrect guesses can get you into trouble.

In this chapter you will learn about three other types of thinking errors. Just like jumping to conclusions, these errors in logic tend to be fueled by your emotions. The goal is to learn enough about thinking errors to be able to catch them when they occur and keep them from affecting your actions in a negative way.

Misperceptions

The first thinking errors to be discussed in this chapter are called misperceptions. They're all about what you do with the information you have. You can distort information in a way that makes you perceive negatives as much bigger and scarier than they really are, or you can discount or reduce positives so that they seem much smaller and less significant than they really are. An example of magnifying the negative might include being late for an appointment and perceiving it as the worst day of your entire life. An example of minimizing a positive might include brushing off a compliment on your appearance because you think you look awful. Magnifying intensifies negative emotions. Minimizing keeps you from enjoying the good feelings that come with positive events or circumstances. These thinking errors often occur when you are in a low or depressed state.

Interestingly, misperceptions can also occur when you are on a high or in a manic phase. In this case, your up mood might make you magnify the positives and minimize the negatives. For example, Miguel recently magnified in his mind how reasonable it was to buy a new Corvette and minimized how upset his wife would be. Miguel's mood swings fluctuate from hypomanic to moderately depressed. He enjoys the highs and doesn't always realize that he is not acting like his usual self. During his last high phase he saw someone driving the new Corvette and decided that he had to have it. In his mind, it was reasonable to trade in the sedan he had recently paid off for a car that he perceived as having better resale value and more power to help him deal with the traffic on the highway. Miguel believed that driving a fast car would improve his mood and reduce his stress, which would make him a better father. So from Miguel's point of view it seemed that a new Corvette would be good for everyone. This is a good example of magnifying the positive. He knew that his wife was happy they had paid off their car because she needed the money for some upcoming family expenses, but he minimized this concern. "She'll fuss for a while, but she'll get over it," he thought. "She always does."

Exercise 10.1 on the next page provides examples of misperceptions in depression. Think of times when you misperceived a situation by either magnifying or minimizing the facts and enter your examples in the spaces provided in the exercise.

Gain Emotional Distance to Control Magnification

In depression and mania, magnification is fueled by the emotion of the moment. When the intensity of the emotion decreases, magnification tends to diminish. For example, if you're angry, an upsetting situation may seem intolerable; once you've calmed down, however, the situation may seem bothersome but manageable. If you're feeling sad and are left out by a group of friends, you might feel devastated at first, but after you are able to calm down you might feel hurt yet able to deal with it. Emotions that fuel magnification can be lessened by gaining emotional distance from an event or idea, allowing you time to think before you react. Exercise 10.2 on page 137 lists some common ways to gain emotional distance. Put a check next to the ones you have tried and any others you are willing to try.

How to Stop Minimizing Positives

There are several different reasons you might tend to minimize positives. When you're not depressed, you might minimize positives or dismiss compliments as an act of humility or

EXERCISE 10.1 Misperceptions in Depression		
Add your own examples next to Amanda's examples of misperceptions.		
Misperception	**Amanda's examples**	**My examples**
Magnification of the seriousness of problems	*This is so horrible. I'll never forgive myself for forgetting my mom's birthday.*	
Minimization of positive events or accomplishments *or* Dismissing compliments	*It doesn't matter that I finally cleaned the kitchen. I should never have let it get this bad.* Amanda's boss: *You did a good job.* Amanda minimizes: *It's no big deal.* Amanda: *Your report card looks pretty good!* Her son minimizes: *Yeah, whatever.*	

modesty. In those situations, pushing away praise is a social behavior, but in your heart you still feel good about the compliment. When in a depressed or irritable state, you might minimize positives because you don't think they count. You might think you're not worthy of praise or your actions are too inadequate to matter. If you have high expectations or are a perfectionist, you might feel that nothing is good enough unless it is perfect. With this train of thought you are not able to enjoy the small accomplishments that build up to become bigger accomplishments. When you're in a bad mood and think that nothing is going your way, you might minimize or completely ignore any evidence to the contrary. Some people minimize positives even when they are not depressed. They can always think of the downside, why things won't work, or what could spoil a positive event. We call them pessimists.

If any of these examples sound like you, then you probably tend to minimize the positives in your life. The downside of doing this is that you miss opportunities to feel good about yourself. Everyone needs emotional boosts on a regular basis. It helps to fight off the emotional impact of the negatives encountered along the way. People who commonly experience low moods claim that they see the world more realistically than others. While it may be true that they don't magnify the positive like those who wear rose-colored glasses, minimizing the positives does not help their depression.

The goal of this chapter is to teach you strategies for dealing with thinking errors. With regard to minimization of positives, you do not have to pretend to be an optimist, you just need to allow yourself the opportunity to see what is right in your world and not just what is wrong with it. The next section provides a strategy to stop minimizing your positives.

THOUGHT STOPPING

To control minimizing, you can use a method called **thought stopping**. This is a strategy that was developed for the treatment of rumination or obsessive thoughts. Its goal is to stop

---

EXERCISE 10.2 Ways to Gain Emotional Distance

Below is a list of strategies for gaining emotional distance. Make a note of the ones you have already tried. Of the ones that remain, select the ones you are willing to try.

Strategies	Things I have tried	Things I am willing to try
Walk away from the situation		
Take time to evaluate it		
Ask others for their opinion of the event		
Sleep on it		
Compare the event that is magnified to other experiences you have had		
Ask yourself how others might view what happened		
Watch television for a while		
Change the subject		
Meditate		
Take a nap		
Refuse to talk about it until you've calmed down		

minimization and replace it with something more accurate. Thought stopping to control minimization involves three steps. Exercise 10.3 will walk you through them.

The first step is to catch yourself doing it. That's the hardest part. It can help to enlist the assistance of someone in your family or a friend to alert you when he or she hears you minimize. Try to pay attention to situations where you become aware of a positive and then push it away. There are probably patterns that you can come to recognize. Maybe your minimization takes the form of dismissing praise, for example. If so, you can watch for it when receiving positive feedback from others. If your pattern is to disqualify things you've accomplished, you probably minimize on a regular basis. As you get things done, listen to that voice in your head that tells you it doesn't count, doesn't matter, or isn't worth mentioning. It can help to keep a log of the types of things you minimize so you can learn to catch yourself in the act of minimizing. Make some notes about these situations in Exercise 10.3A.

EXERCISE 10.3A **Thought Stopping Step 1: Identify Triggers**	
In the space below, make a note of situations where you tend to minimize positives and write down what you tend to say to yourself or others. An example has been provided.	
Situations where I minimize positives	**What I say to myself or others**
When people compliment me on how I look.	*I say thank you, but what I really think is that I've gained weight and look awful. They complimented me because they noticed that I'm fat and didn't know what else to say.*

EXERCISE 10.3B Thought Stopping Step 2: Stop Command	
Write down some words you can say to yourself when you minimize positives. Use the triggers you listed in the last exercise to come up with an appropriate statement.	
Situations where I minimize the positives	**My STOP command**
When people compliment me on how I look.	Don't say it! Take the compliment!

The second step is to control the thought by telling yourself in a commanding voice to "STOP!" Practice telling yourself to "STOP!" You may not be able to say it aloud, but you can think it to yourself. Find a tone of voice that sounds like an authority, like a parent. "Stop saying that!" "Don't push away the compliment!" "Cut that out!" Think about how you would tell someone else in a strong voice to stop an annoying behavior. Use that tone on yourself when you catch yourself minimizing your positives. Take a moment to come up with an example and write it down in Exercise 10.3B above.

The third step is to switch the thought to something more positive. If you catch yourself about to dismiss a compliment from someone, tell yourself to "STOP!" and say "Thank you" instead. If you catch yourself minimizing your accomplishments, like getting some work done that might have been hard for you, tell yourself that it's OK to feel good about it. Try statements like "Doing something is better than doing nothing" or "It may be a small accomplishment, but it's still positive" or "When I'm feeling this bad, anything I can do is a good thing." You will have to find a thought to replace your minimization. The most helpful ones are those that allow you to see your positives for what they are. Give this some thought and jot down your more positive responses in Exercise 10.3C on the next page.

Raquel had a bad habit of pushing away praise and telling herself that even when she did do something right, it wasn't good enough. She learned to use thought stopping to control her minimization. The most common example for Raquel is that when people praised her, she followed their compliments with self-criticism. For example, an interaction with her best friend might have sounded like this:

EXERCISE 10.3C Thought Stopping Step 3: Positive Alternatives	
Write down some positive alternatives to minimizing positive statements. Make it a point to practice them when you have the urge to minimize.	
Situations where I minimize the positives	**My positive response**
When people compliment me on how I look.	I will say thank you and nothing else.

BEST FRIEND: You look great in that dress. [praise]

RAQUEL: It's too tight in the hips. [self-criticism]

BEST FRIEND: You look fine. [praise]

RAQUEL: Your standards are too low. [discounted her praise]

The end result of many conversations like this was that compliments were delivered but never received by Raquel. Therefore, they had no positive impact on her. Rejection of compliments frustrated Raquel's best friend, so after a while she learned not to offer them anymore. Raquel noticed at some point that her friend had stopped praising her. Her interpretation was that she must really look fat because her friend had stopped pretending that she looked fine. One year, Raquel worked particularly hard to lose weight before their class reunion. At the event, Raquel received praise about how she looked from everyone except her best friend. She took offense and acted coldly toward her until her friend got irritated with her and asked, "Why are you acting that way?" When she told her friend what had upset her, the friend explained that she had given up trying to praise Raquel's appearance because it seemed like compliments upset her rather than making her feel good about herself.

Raquel got some therapy for the depression and learned thought stopping. One of the problems she learned to control was her tendency to have unrealistic standards for herself and others. Rejecting praise (minimizing positives from others) was just one of the many ways that it showed. She made improvements, and now when someone compliments her appearance she tells herself to "STOP!" before the negative remark leaves her lips. Her new response is "Thank you. You are very kind."

Tunnel Vision

Tunnel vision is another type of thinking error. It has to do with the tendency to see only the things that confirm your point of view and ignore or disregard information to the contrary. This thinking error can occur when your mood is up as well as when it is down. Here's an example. When Amanda is depressed, she is convinced that she's a loser. She remembers the mistakes she has made, the decisions she regrets, and the goals that she never met. Focusing attention on the things that confirm your view is part of tunnel vision. In addition, Amanda ignores any information that is contrary to her negative view. She overlooks, forgets, or refuses to acknowledge her successes, her strengths, and the times things worked out OK for her. Ignoring contrary evidence is the second aspect of tunnel vision. It's like looking through a lens that allows you to see only what is directly in front of you and failing to see everything else around you.

Tunnel vision in mania is similar. When your mood swings upward, you may see evidence that confirms your positive or overly optimistic view and ignore evidence against it even when people disagree with you. An example might include seeing a risky investment opportunity as being a sure bet even though your friends and family say you are being misled or manipulated by others.

Stan gets paranoid when he is having a manic episode. He thinks people at work are against him. What Stan does not see is that when he is paranoid and fearful he acts differently toward people at work. His suspiciousness shows. He is guarded, communicates less with others, and accuses them of touching things on this desk, being mean to him, or failing to keep him informed. When Stan is like this, people tend to stay away from him. He is unpleasant, and the change from his usual jovial self is confusing. No one knows that he has bipolar disorder, although they suspect that something is wrong with him. Their changes in behavior toward Stan confirm his paranoia.

The part that Stan forgets, does not see, or ignores is the evidence that people at work generally like him. He also forgets that when he is becoming manic he does not trust people. This is why tunnel vision can be hard to fix. In the moment, you are convinced that your view is accurate. It feels right. To overcome tunnel vision you have to be able to slow down and think it through, listen to the views of others, know yourself well enough to know that you sometimes have tunnel vision, and consider the possibility that it is distorting your view of yourself, of other people, and of your future.

How to Get Out of the Tunnel

COPING WITH NEGATIVE TUNNEL VISION

The way out of tunnel vision is to force yourself to look at the big picture. You have to make yourself examine all available information before you draw a conclusion. Look at the good news and the bad news, the evidence that your idea is right and that it is wrong, and then decide what to think. If you are feeling down and engaged in negative tunnel vision, you are probably missing the situations in which:

- Things have gone right
- Problems have been solved effectively
- People were kind to you
- You received positive feedback
- You were able to take action

One way to protect yourself from tunnel vision is to keep a running list of these positive experiences. Miguel, for example, has a tendency to be critical of himself when he is feeling depressed. During those times he thinks he is worthless, and the more he dwells on it the worse he feels. To protect himself from tunnel vision, Miguel keeps a list of his successes on his smartphone. Every time things go right, he is able to solve an important problem, or he makes it through a difficult time in his life, he makes a note of the event. When he is feeling low and his focus turns to self-doubt, he reviews his list. Because the list is written in his own words, it is more powerful than the reassuring words of his family members. They try to encourage Miguel, but he minimizes their positive words and argues back with a list of his failures. In contrast, when he reads his own list of successes he remembers when he wrote them and how good it felt to do something right. This is Miguel's strategy for fighting negative tunnel vision. When his wife can't get through to him, she says, "If you don't believe me, just read your list." He may not do it right away, but her reminder eventually gets him to review his successes, and when he does, he begins to feel better about himself. Start your list in Exercise 10.4 on the facing page.

DON'T BE MISLED BY POSITIVE TUNNEL VISION

Positive tunnel vision can occur during upswings in your mood due to hypomania or mania. It is the tendency to try to convince yourself or others that everything is fine, that all things will work out, or that there's nothing to worry about even when there is plenty of evidence that this isn't true. It is not just about trying to kid yourself. During positive mood swings, tunnel vision may keep you from seeing:

- The times you were wrong
- Mistakes in judgment that caused you problems
- Periods when too much optimism clouded your thinking
- Signs that you are getting manic
- The risks involved in your choices

One of the easiest ways to protect yourself from tunnel vision is to share your ideas with someone you trust. This should be a person who knows about your mood swings and has nothing to gain or lose by your decisions. Therapists can serve this function, but if you are not in therapy you can choose someone else like your AA sponsor, a close friend, a member of the clergy, or someone from a support group you belong to, like the Depression and Bipolar

EXERCISE 10.4 **Things You've Done Right**

Make a list of things you have done right. Use it to remind yourself of your successes when your tunnel vision lets you see only the negatives. Put this list on your smartphone or computer, or in your work space. Read it regularly.

Things I have done well, accomplishments, and successes.

Times I have been able to overcome problems, persevere, or not give up.

Times I thought I would fail but didn't.

Difficulties I resolved.

Support Alliance (*www.dbsalliance.org*). The easy part is getting advice from others. The hard part is having the self-awareness that you need advice. If your symptoms of hypomania or mania are already severe, you may not realize that you have tunnel vision until it is too late and you have impulsively acted on a manic idea. If that happens, try to learn from the experience. Make a note to ask a neutral party the next time someone close to you challenges your positive tunnel vision.

All-or-Nothing Thinking

It is easy to spot all-or-nothing thinking in other people. They use words that give away their view. They label people or events in absolute terms such as:

- "She is absolutely useless."
- "No one understands me."
- "You are either for me or against me."
- "I will never take medication."

Seeing yourself as either a success or a failure, seeing others as either good or bad, and believing that there is only one right way to do things usually come with stress, disappointment, and hopelessness. There is no middle ground with these types of statements—they are inflexible, uncompromising, and perfectionistic. And most important, it is hard to imagine a way to fix these things. There is not much you can do about them.

In reality, things in life are rarely at the positive or negative extremes. Most of the time things are somewhere in the middle. Here are some examples of the same general ideas without the all-or-nothing language. They are more specific and therefore open the door to possible solutions. Compare them to the ones on page 143.

- "She is useless only when it comes to being on time."
- "A few people understand me, but my mother doesn't, and that irritates me."
- "I want you to be for me, but right now it seems like you are against me."
- "I don't like being sick."
- "I don't like the idea of having to take medication. I want to find another way first."

When you read these two sets of statements, can you feel the difference? This second set is more forgiving, allows room for compromise, and expresses preferences and feelings rather than condemning others or declaring inflexible positions. You can imagine solutions like letting someone know how important it is to you that she be on time, communicating more with your mother so that she understands you better, letting others know that you need their support, or expressing your distress about your illness and your preference not to take medication for it.

How to Control All-or-Nothing Thinking

The goal here is not to become a positive thinker. The goal is to be more accurate, more precise with your words and your thoughts. Frame your problems or complaints in a way that leads you to some possible solutions. The trick is to remove the distortions so you can more clearly see what needs to be fixed. Start with trying to recognize all-or-nothing thoughts by the extreme words you think and say. Exercise 10.5 on the facing page includes a list of words and phrases that are typical of all-or-nothing thinking. Jot down an example of how you might use these words or phrases. If you are uncertain, listen to yourself for a few days or ask a close friend or family member if he or she has ever heard you use these words.

The next step is to change your thinking from all-or-nothing to a more accurate view. For example, instead of saying "Everyone thinks I'm a loser," make the statement more factually accurate, such as "I'm worried that my wife thinks I am a loser because I lost my job." This more precise version opens the door to an intervention—talk to your wife about your worry. Give her a chance to speak for herself.

Review the examples you provided in Exercise 10.5 and try to revise your statements so that they are more specific and more accurately express how you feel. Try to think of what can be done to solve the problem. Exercise 10.6 on page 146 provides some examples.

EXERCISE 10.5 Examples of All-or-Nothing Words and Phrases

Extreme word/phrase	Examples	Your personal example
No one	No one cares about this house except me.	
Never	We never do what I want to do.	
Always	You always criticize me.	
Everyone	Everyone thinks I'm a loser.	
Can't	I can't do anything about it.	
Absolutely	This is absolutely ridiculous.	
Should	I shouldn't make mistakes.	
Labels	She is so stupid!	

What's Next?

The exercises in this workbook have emphasized the connections between how you think and how you feel. Negative thoughts can leave you with negative feelings that fuel negative mood swings. If you can learn to recognize common errors in your logic, you will be able to replace your overly negative thoughts with more logical ones. Logical thoughts are those that help you see a situation more clearly. If you can't tell the difference between an emotional thought and a logical thought, the exercises in the next chapter will help you figure it out. Seeing things more clearly is an important step toward reducing your negative feelings, solving problems, and improving your self-esteem.

EXERCISE 10.6 How to Make All-or-Nothing Thoughts More Specific		
Extreme word/phrase	**Examples**	**More specific thoughts and plans**
No one	No one cares about this house except me.	The kids are making a mess, and I am doing the housework. I need to get them to help.
Never	We never do what I want to do.	I usually let my friends choose where we go to dinner. I need to speak up about where I want to go.
Always	You always criticize me.	I don't like it when my boss criticizes me. It hurts my feelings. I need to let him know and ask for some positive feedback too.
Everyone	Everyone thinks I'm a loser.	I'm worried that my wife thinks I am a loser because I lost my job. I need to talk to her about this.
Can't	I can't do anything about it.	I feel helpless sometimes. I don't know what to do. I need some help.
Absolutely	Absolutely not!	I do not want to do things your way. Let's try to find a compromise.
Should	I shouldn't make mistakes.	I don't like making mistakes. It is embarrassing. I will be more careful next time.
Labels	She is so stupid!	I don't agree with what she said. I can tell her if the topic is important to me.

11

Analyze Your Thoughts

In this chapter you will:

✓ Develop new skills to control negative emotions.

✓ Learn how to tell the difference between logical and emotional thoughts.

✓ Find out how to use thought records to analyze negative thoughts.

Thought Records

In Chapters 7 and 10 you learned about common thinking errors and what you can do to fight them off. Sometimes, however, it's not obvious whether your thoughts are accurate or distorted by emotion, especially when stressful things happen. An upsetting or stimulating event can leave you feeling overwhelmed by many different negative thoughts and feelings at the same time. A thought record is a tool for sorting it all out. Once you have a clearer picture of what is going on, you can come up with a plan for how to proceed.

There are several advantages of using a thought record. It's easier to write down your thoughts before trying to analyze or change them instead of trying to do it all in your head. Emotions make it hard to think. Putting your thoughts on paper slows down the process and gives you time to work things out. If you have several thoughts at one time, writing them out allows you to work on one thought at a time. In addition, seeing your thoughts on paper can help you more quickly identify errors in logic. It's easy to believe that distorted thoughts are true until you see them in writing. Also, certain types of emotion-filled thoughts tend to recur, like the thinking errors described in Chapters 7 and 10. If you keep your thought records, you can refer back to your notes and more quickly work through new problems or emotional situations. Another advantage is that if you want to share your work with your doctor or therapist, it is easier to provide the thought record than to try to recall an upsetting event and the thoughts and feelings you had at the time.

Thought records usually have two parts—one part for recording your thoughts and one part for analyzing your thoughts. Exercise 11.1 below is the first part of a thought record; it helps you record your thoughts about upsetting events. It includes a place to describe the event that triggered a strong emotional reaction and the thoughts and feelings that followed. There isn't always a specific event that sets off an emotional reaction, but if there is one, recording the event will help you learn about the types of events that might set you off in the future. You may download and print additional copies of this thought record from *www. guilford.com/basco2-forms* and add them to your workbook as needed.

Paul's thought record shows that he got upset when his girlfriend did not return his phone call. He didn't know why she hadn't called, but he imagined the worst. He used his thought record to try to calm himself because the longer he waited for her call, the more he imagined the worst. His worry fueled his self-blame and catastrophizing, as can be seen by the thoughts and feelings he recorded.

EXERCISE 11.1 Thought Record, Part I		
Event What triggered your thoughts and feelings?	**Thoughts** Write down all the thoughts that popped into your mind when the event occurred.	**Feelings** What feelings did you experience? Include emotions and physical sensations.

From *The Bipolar Workbook, Second Edition.* Copyright 2015 by The Guilford Press.

PAUL'S EXAMPLE Thought Record, Part I		
Event	**Thoughts**	**Feelings**
Girlfriend did not return phone call	She must be mad at me. She doesn't want to talk to me.	Sadness
	It's my fault for not returning her call right away last time.	Guilt
	I'm such a lousy boyfriend.	Guilt
	I bet she's going to dump me.	Grief

Use Exercise 11.1 (Thought Record, Part I) to record a recent event that caused you a lot of distress. See if you can recall your thoughts and the feelings that went along with them. If you can't think of a prior event, wait until something happens to upset you and then try to record your thought about the event.

Evaluating Your Thoughts

The immediate thoughts you have in response to an event might be overly negative or overly positive. Sometimes these will be distortions, and sometimes these thoughts will be accurate. If you're not certain whether your thoughts are true or false, you will need to put them to a test. Here are some ways to test your thoughts for accuracy.

Ways to Evaluate the Accuracy of Your Thoughts

There are a number of strategies you can use to evaluate your emotion-filled thoughts. You use your own strategies every time you stop to think about a situation before you draw a conclusion about it. You usually don't need an exercise or worksheet to figure it out. However, when you feel stuck or overwhelmed by strong feelings, it can help to have some step-by-step procedures for pulling yourself out of it. When it comes to addressing emotional thoughts, the procedures help you step back from the emotion a little and use your logic to reason through the problem.

For example, you might try looking back through your personal examples of thinking errors from Chapters 7 and 10 to see if the thoughts you listed in your thought record fall under one of those categories. If so, follow the instructions in those chapters for correcting those thinking errors. Another simple strategy is to ask people for their opinions. Do the people you trust see things the same way that you do, or do they think you are being overly positive or overly negative? Both strategies are ways of gathering information to help you make an informed decision about the situation that is troubling you. You will have to draw your own conclusion, but gathering information will help you be objective rather than rely only on your emotions or gut feelings to guide you.

LOGICAL ANALYSIS OF EMOTIONAL THOUGHTS

The second part of the thought record guides you through several exercises for analyzing your thoughts and drawing objective conclusions. The hope is that when you are able to see things clearly, without distortion that can be fueled by emotion, you can deal more effectively with the problem. Exercise 11.2 on the facing page includes key questions that challenge you to be logical when you are faced with an upsetting event. One way to use it is to pick the thought from Part I of the thought record that is most upsetting to you or that is associated with the most emotion. Write that thought at the top of Exercise 11.2 on page 151. Before you begin analyzing the thought, take a moment to ask yourself how strongly you believe it. Are you 100% convinced that it is true, or do you have some doubt? A rating of 50% would mean that you could go either way, and 10% would mean that you don't really believe it at all. If your rating is low then you may not need Exercise 11.2. You may have already done an analysis of the facts in your head and have already drawn a conclusion. What is left for you to figure out is whether there is anything you need to do about the situation.

To use Part II of the thought record to logically analyze your thoughts, start with the first two columns. In the first column, fill in any facts that support your thought, and in the second column fill in any facts that are contrary to your thought. Try to be as objective as you can. List only factual information, things that can be verified or observed. Do not include your opinion as evidence, such as "I just don't think I'm wrong." Keep in mind that it will always be easier to find evidence that supports an emotional or negative view than evidence against it. You will have to work harder and take more time to come up with evidence against an idea that you "feel" is accurate.

If you have difficulty coming up with factual evidence for or against your upsetting or emotional thought, try using the third column to consider other points of view. For example, what would someone else say in your situation? Write down a few examples. After you have some time to think about it, try to draw a conclusion that makes the most sense. If you find it difficult, ask someone you trust for his or her opinion.

In the fourth column, write down your conclusion. If you find that after giving it some thought you are less convinced that your original thought was true, change your original thought to make it more accurate and more believable. Whatever your conclusion, make a few notes about what you need to do about the situation. You may download and print additional copies of this thought record from *www.guilford.com/basco2-forms* and add them to your workbook as needed.

Amanda provides a good example of how to think through a stressful situation by testing out the validity of some negative thoughts that were stirred up by an upsetting event. She received a notice in the mail that it was time for her to renew her nursing license. The new application had a place for reporting whether or not she had been treated or is being treated for a mental illness. This was a new part of the application since the last time she

EXERCISE 11.2	Thought Record, Part II: Logical Analysis of Thoughts

My thought is:

How strongly do I believe it? _____ (0% = not at all; 100% = believe it completely)

What evidence do I have that my thought is true?	What evidence do I have that my thought is not true?	What would someone else say in this situation?	My conclusions and my plan for what to do next

had renewed her license. No one in nursing knew that Amanda had bipolar disorder, and she did not want to have to tell anyone. She was very upset about the implications of this new rule. She wrote down her immediate thoughts on the thought record below to try to get her bearings on the situation.

All of Amanda's thoughts fall into the category of jumping to conclusions. She noticed this but was still not convinced that the thoughts were false. What fuels her fears is mistrust of her boss, of her coworkers, and of the state nursing board. Even when Amanda is not upset, she thinks that her boss, coworkers, and the nurses on the state board try to appear supportive but are capable of stabbing her in the back. Her instinct is to lie on her application or to refuse to complete that item even though both of those options could have negative consequences. Her immediate course of action was to avoid sending in her renewal application for as long as possible.

After completing the thought record, Amanda picked the thought that bothered her most and tried to analyze it (see p. 153).

AMANDA'S EXAMPLE Thought Record, Part I

Event What triggered your thoughts and feelings?	**Thoughts** Write down all the thoughts that popped into your mind when the event occurred.	**Feelings** What feelings did you experience? Include emotions and physical sensations.
Finding out that I would have to report that I had bipolar disorder to the nursing board	This is horrible. They are not going to renew my license. I will be out of work. We are not going to be able to pay our bills.	Fear
	The nursing board is going to have to tell my employer, and everyone at work will know that I have bipolar disorder.	Anger Frustration
	When my boss finds out, she is going to think that I can't take care of patients. She will watch me like a hawk and find a reason to fire me.	Anger Fear
	My boss will tell others, and I will be completely humiliated.	Embarrassment

AMANDA'S EXAMPLE Thought Record, Part II: Logical Analysis of Thoughts

Amanda's thought: They are not going to renew my license. I will be out of work. We are not going to be able to pay our bills.

What evidence do I have that my thought is true?	What evidence do I have that my thought is not true?	What would someone else say in this situation?	My conclusions and my plan for what to do next
If you do not have a license, you cannot practice nursing in a hospital. Licenses are checked every year. There has been a trend in recent years of reprimanding nurses with substance abuse problems. Those who have lost their licenses are listed in the state board bulletin each year. Many nurses will not take medication for depression because they are afraid of losing their jobs.	The application does not say that I will lose my license. I haven't heard of anyone other than those with substance abuse problems losing their licenses. It would be discrimination to take away your license just because you've been in treatment. There are laws against that. My husband says that I can't lose my license over this.	Someone else would say that I won't know unless I ask. My husband says it's just a bureaucratic maneuver. The nursing board is not going to put itself at risk of getting sued by a bunch of nurses. They can't violate your privacy by telling your boss about your illness.	Find a way to anonymously ask about the rules. Find out what the consequences would be if I lied about my illness. Find out if and how the board will check on the truthfulness of answers to questions about mental illness. If I find out that the board is going to take action on my license, hire a lawyer to help me with this. Renew my application on time. Don't delay it and draw attention to my case.

When you look at evidence for and against a thought, you have to take into consideration the importance of each piece of evidence before you draw any conclusions. It's possible that one column will have a lot more evidence than the other. This does not necessarily mean that the column with more items is more valid. You have to take into consideration how much each item influences your belief in the idea you're testing.

Amanda knows that what makes her fear most believable is that other nurses have said they won't take medications or see a counselor when they need one because they're afraid of losing their jobs. On the opposite side of the argument, what makes her worry less is that she trusts her husband's judgment. Ultimately, she will have to get more information about this new reporting rule before she will feel any relief.

Amanda made a plan to get as much information as she could before she turned in her renewal application. She will start with a nurse she knows at a different hospital. Sally is older than Amanda and also has bipolar disorder. Sally keeps up on the state board rules and may be able to address Amanda's concerns. If she doesn't know, Sally will know whom to ask without getting into trouble.

Amanda considered quitting her job and letting her license expire but decided it would be better to be let go than to leave voluntarily. She did not want to make it easy for them to discriminate against her.

Amanda analyzed each of her worries on the thought record using the methods described. Working through her thoughts in a systematic way did not take away all of Amanda's anxiety or anger, but it did help her calm down enough to come up with a reasonable plan for dealing with her problem.

Tommy is learning to use thought records to cope with the ideas he gets when he is becoming manic. The last few times he got manic, he had the urge to take a trip. One time he got in his car and drove until he ran out of gas. He had forgotten his wallet, so he had to call his mom to come bring him gasoline. She refused to let him drive his car, so he had to go home with her. Another time, he bought a round-trip ticket to Hawaii on a credit card his father had given him to use for school expenses. He left without telling anyone where he was going. He hung out at the beach for a few days but did not have any fun. When he came back, his parents were furious and canceled his credit card. Tommy practiced with his therapist how to analyze his urges to travel before he goes on the road.

When the urge to leave town hits him, Tommy always gets the idea that he has to follow his instinct or he'll go crazy. Every minute he waits feels like an eternity. He also tends to have the idea that everything will turn out fine if he goes. There will be no negative consequences, only relief from the pressure he feels. During a therapy visit, when the urge to travel was only mild, Tommy and his therapist worked through the steps to analyze these thoughts (see the facing page).

After you've completed your thought record and thought analysis, go back and examine your original thoughts. Can you see how being objective changes your thoughts? What did you notice about the intensity of the emotions you originally felt? If your emotions are still pretty intense, try one of the other methods mentioned in this chapter or in Chapters 7 and 10 for coping with your emotional thoughts.

TOMMY'S EXAMPLE	Thought Record, Part I	
Event What triggered your thoughts and feelings?	**Thoughts** Write down all the thoughts that popped into your mind when the event occurred.	**Feelings** What feelings did you experience? Include emotions and physical sensations.
Got the urge to go to Hawaii	I want to go to Hawaii this weekend. I need to get away from the cold weather. It's a good idea.	Excited
	I will feel better if I go to Hawaii.	Excited
	I don't care about the money. I deserve a break.	Confident
	If I don't get out of town, I'm going to go crazy.	Stressed

TOMMY'S EXAMPLE	Thought Record, Part II: Logical Analysis of Thoughts		
Tommy's thought: *If I don't get out of town, I'm going to go crazy.*			
What evidence do I have that my thought is true?	**What evidence do I have that my thought is not true?**	**What would someone else say in this situation?**	**My conclusions and my plan for what to do next**
I can feel myself getting more uptight each day. I can't stand being in my apartment every day. I hate the cold weather. I always feel better when I'm at the beach.	No one actually goes crazy because they can't travel. I've felt this way before. The urge eventually goes away.	My mother would say that I'm manic again. My father would probably agree. It is the middle of the semester, and if I miss any more classes, I will probably fail them.	I will plan a trip to Hawaii during spring break if I still have the urge to go by then. I'll do other things to control my restless feelings. I will take the medication the doctor gave me and work out at the gym more often.

"I CAN'T DO IT."

If you are a black-and-white thinker like Amanda and the exercise you're trying doesn't make you feel better right away, you may give up on it too easily. Progress may be noticeable but small at first. For example, if you're trying to combat the negative thought "I'm stupid," after evaluating the evidence you may be partially but not completely convinced that you were wrong about yourself. If you have held on to a negative view of yourself for a long time, it will take some work to convince yourself otherwise. You have to retrain your thought process by continually practicing methods for evaluating and correcting your overly negative ideas. With practice, change can become permanent. So if you find yourself thinking "I can't do it" and feeling frustrated, take a break and then try again, because giving up too soon will only reinforce your negative thoughts.

What's Next?

This chapter introduced you to thought records. This is a commonly used exercise in cognitive-behavioral therapy. Therapists usually give thought records as homework assignments and ask people to write down thoughts associated with upsetting events that might occur between therapy sessions. You can do the same for yourself. When you experience an event that upsets you, work through the first part of the thought record to try to identify what bothers you the most and use the second part to reason through your logic. Many people find this very helpful. With regular practice you may find that you can work through the logic of your negative thoughts without having to write anything down. Some of what you learned in this chapter will help you work through any negative feelings about taking medications for your mood swings. Chapter 12 uses similar strategies to help you get the most out of your medication.

12

Work through Denial about Needing Medication

In this chapter you will:

✓ Discover how people make the adjustment to having bipolar disorder.

✓ Find out how this workbook can help you come to terms with the illness.

✓ Learn the basic facts about medication treatment for bipolar disorder.

Tommy, Paul, Amanda, Miguel, and Raquel have all gone through times in their lives when they did not take prescribed medication for their symptoms of bipolar disorder. When Tommy was first diagnosed, he did not believe he had it. While he was in the hospital, he took medication as he was told, but as soon as he was back in his apartment on his own he stopped taking it. His parents would ask him about his medications because they could see that he was still not acting like his old self. Tommy would lie and say that he was taking it, and his parents would believe him. Within a few weeks Tommy would be manic again and would have to be hospitalized. Tommy was hospitalized four times within 7 months, with each hospitalization increasing in length. He is still young, and he has not gone off his medication since his last hospitalization. But there will be challenges ahead when he may take himself off medications again to see what will happen.

Paul started taking medication for bipolar disorder when he was just a kid. Acceptance of his diagnosis was never a question. His parents told him what he had and gave him medicine for it. He took it regularly until he was in middle school. From eighth grade to his junior year of high school, Paul and his parents were constantly debating about his medications. Paul no longer accepted their directions about lots of things, including taking medication. He rebelled and refused to take it for months at a time. What would bring him back to treatment was having a severe period of depression. It always took medication to get him out of it. In his junior year of high school he got drunk and tried to kill himself. He ran his car into a tree and suffered many injuries. Surgery, physical therapy, and medication brought him back to normal. Paul did not want to go to those depths of depression again, and he had learned that going off medication meant that depression would eventually return.

Amanda really hates the idea of taking medication because it reminds her that she has bipolar disorder and is "not normal." Because she knows she is stuck with this illness forever, she goes through periods of being very angry about it, especially when it seems to be disrupting her life or keeping her from reaching her goals. During those times she tinkers with her medication regimen, trying to make the medicine more tolerable to take. When her symptoms get too severe for her to handle on her own, she calls her doctor for help. She has received numerous lectures from doctors over the years about not taking her medications consistently, waiting until the last minute to call for help, and not coming to grips with having bipolar disorder. Amanda has usually responded to those lectures by changing doctors and repeating the pattern once again.

Miguel has bipolar II disorder. He has had several very severe episodes of major depression, but he has never had full manic episodes. Even though he gets pretty hypomanic at times, it has never caused him any serious or life-threatening problems. It has hurt his family, gotten him into jail, and caused him to lose a few jobs. In his youth, his excuse had always been that he was young and needed to grow up. This made it easy for Miguel to pretend that his highs were not a problem. Miguel's last severe episode of depression occurred when he was in his early 20s and lasted for several months. He was not suicidal, but he had lost all desire to work, spend time with this family, or see his friends. His parents pressured him to seek treatment and ultimately threatened to kick him out of their house if he did not agree to see a psychiatrist. It worked, but when his psychiatrist tried to give him a mood stabilizer, Miguel refused to take it. He agreed to take an antidepressant medication because he knew he had problems with depression, but he would not accept a diagnosis of bipolar II disorder. Unfortunately, taking antidepressants sometimes worsens his mood swings. Miguel is older now and sees himself as wiser. However, he has not fully accepted that his highs can cause as much trouble as his lows.

DABDA

Each of the individuals described in this workbook has struggled with the psychological and emotional burden not only of having to deal with life-altering mood swings, but also of being diagnosed with a mood disorder that requires ongoing medication treatment. Coping with the emotional adjustment takes place in phases, similar to the phases that people go through when they are grieving—denial, anger, bargaining, depression, and acceptance (DABDA). There is an initial period of denial and disbelief. When the person with the illness is a child, it can be the parents who are in denial. This is sometimes followed by misdirected anger at the doctor, at the person with the symptoms, at God for allowing it to happen, or at other people who are blamed, such as the parent who passed on the genes for a mood disorder. Denial and anger can fluctuate back and forth and can even return after you thought you had adjusted to the diagnosis, the illness, and the treatment. The emotions usually resurface when the mood swings recur and disrupt your life.

Bargaining is another one of those phases that people experience when they are adjusting to bad news. People who have not yet accepted their diagnosis of bipolar disorder or a related illness that causes mood swings will make secret deals with themselves such as promising to stop drinking or using street drugs, to start a diet, see a therapist, or begin an exercise regimen. They think these things will stabilize their mood so that medication will not be needed. Because mood swings recur, their plan usually works for only a short time, until the symptoms cycle back around.

Once a person has accepted the reality of having chronic mood swings it is not unusual to become very distressed and even depressed about it. When the full weight of what it means to have a chronic mental illness that will not go away sinks in, it can be overwhelming. With time and support, this feeling will dissipate, and you can take charge of doing whatever you can to feel better. If you bought this workbook for yourself, you must be past the denial stage and are working your way to acceptance. If someone gave it to you, perhaps you need some more information and more time to adjust to the idea. The information in the first few chapters of this workbook was intended to help you understand the symptoms. If you identified with what you read, your denial may be lessening already.

This workbook was intended for people with mood swings caused by a variety of problems. If you are not yet certain about your diagnosis or the need for medication, perhaps you can focus your energy on learning as much as you can about how to control your mood swings while you continue to investigate the causes and the treatments.

Where are you in your stages of adjustment to a diagnosis of bipolar disorder or another disorder associated with mood swings? Exercise 12.1 provides some examples of the kinds of thoughts and actions that accompany each stage of adjustment. Read through the examples and try to identify where you fit.

What to Do Next

There are exercises in this workbook that may help you with your adjustment. The following exercises match the stages of adjustment with the chapters that introduce skills that may help you come to terms with your diagnosis (see pp. 160 and 161). If you are uncertain about the underlying causes of your mood swings and feel hesitant about treatment, talk it over with an expert such as a psychiatrist, social worker, psychologist, counselor, or psychiatric nurse practitioner.

EXERCISE 12.1	**Where Are You in the Stages of Adjustment to Bipolar Disorder?**

Circle the automatic thoughts and actions that best describe where you are in your adjustment.

Stage	Automatic thoughts	Actions
Denial	*I don't have it. The doctor made a mistake.* *It must be because I've been drinking too much.* *The diagnosis is wrong.*	Getting a second opinion Looking for other explanations for symptoms Ignoring treatment recommendations
Anger	*It's not fair that I have this illness.* *I can't deal with this right now.* *Why me? What did I do to deserve this?*	Refusing to listen to advice Refusing to discuss the illness Losing temper with health care providers, pharmacies, or anyone else associated with treatment
Bargaining	*I'll clean up my act.* *I'll stop drinking, start waking up on time, start exercising, get a better job, and it will be OK.* *I'll try natural remedies. I don't really need medicine.*	Adjusting doses on your own Changing the timing of doses Trading active drugs for "natural remedies" Staying up late to avoid taking sleeping medications Drinking alcohol to reduce anxiety
Depression	*I'll never have a normal life.* *No one will want me.* *I hate myself.*	Self-destructive behaviors Avoidance of stimuli related to the illness Withdrawal from others
Acceptance	*I can work my way through this.* *It's not the end of the world.* *I don't have to give up everything just because I have to take medication.*	Adherence to treatment Open discussion of treatment options with clinicians before discontinuing medications

	Helpful Chapters for Each Stage of Adjustment	
Stage	**Indicators**	**Chapter**
Denial	You do not trust the diagnosis and are not ready to take medication.	Chapter 1 explains why medication is needed to control mood symptoms and Chapters 2 and 3 describe common symptoms of bipolar disorder. The remainder of this chapter and Chapter 13 will explain why it's important to take medication consistently.
Anger	Anger at having a psychiatric diagnosis keeps you from using good coping strategies.	Chapter 7 can teach you how not to let your emotions override your logic.
Bargaining	You know you have a problem. You are willing to stop some unhealthy habits and replace them with some healthier habits to try to control your symptoms.	Chapter 5 can help you identify factors that trigger mood swings, and Chapter 6 can teach you how to avoid things that make symptoms worse.
Depression	You are aware that you have bipolar disorder, and you find it depressing.	Chapter 8 will help you get unstuck and take some action. Chapters 10 and 11 will help you cope with depressing thoughts.
Acceptance	You are ready to do what you can to control your mood swings.	Chapter 13 will help you be consistent in taking your medications. Chapters 14 through 17 will show you how to strengthen your coping skills.

Basic Facts about Medication Treatment for Bipolar Disorder

If you've been diagnosed with bipolar disorder, more than likely you have been prescribed medication to control your symptoms. Taking medications for this illness is not like taking medications for a cold or an infection or to control pain. Following are some basic facts about the medication treatment of bipolar disorder.

• **Fact 1: Medication is required to fully control the symptoms of this disorder and to prevent symptoms from returning once they have remitted.** A significant amount of research has been conducted on the treatment of depression and mania in bipolar disorder, and the results consistently show that people tend to do better with medication than without it.

• **Fact 2: Most people who have bipolar disorder do not like taking medication. And most go through periods of time when they stop it altogether, take it less consistently, or alter the regimen on their own to try to make it more tolerable.** The research on adherence to treatment for bipolar disorder shows that the majority of people with bipolar disorder take some of their medications most of the time and all of their medications some of the time. A smaller group of people take all their medications all of the time, particularly those who are organized and consistent about other things in their lives. And there are some people who stop taking all of their medications altogether. Over your lifetime of dealing with bipolar disorder there is a good chance that you will have times when you take less medication than your doctor would prefer or take it less consistently than prescribed.

• **Fact 3: Most medications prescribed for the symptoms of bipolar disorder do not work unless they are taken very consistently and at a dose high enough to have a positive effect.** This may sound obvious, but because the mood swings come and go, it's easy to assume that medication can be used off and on.

Tommy challenged his doctor when he insisted that Tommy keep taking Depakote and lithium even after his mania subsided.

"I don't see why I have to. I had strep throat last year that got really bad. I had to be on two different antibiotics to finally kill it. But when the infection was gone, I didn't need to keep taking more antibiotics just to keep from ever getting another one. So why should I keep taking lithium? It makes me tired. I can hardly concentrate in class, and I'm not manic anymore."

Tommy made an interesting point that on the surface does not sound illogical. Tommy's doctor explained that bipolar disorder is not an infection or virus that goes away. The medications control the symptoms and can help to keep mania and depression from returning, but they do not fix the underlying biological problem that produces the symptoms. It's similar to having diabetes in this way. People take medication to control the symptoms of diabetes, but so far there is no real cure.

Tommy has been told this before and seems to understand the concept but is not ready to fully accept the idea that he has a chronic mental illness. He went along with treatment while he was feeling bad, but he never envisioned having to take medication for the rest of his life.

• **Fact 4: Taking medication daily for bipolar disorder is not just about the pills; it is about accepting a fate you may not be ready to take on.** Amanda still struggles with this idea. The intellectual side of her understands that she has an illness that requires treatment. She is tired of struggling against the illness and against the doctors and really wants to have more stability in her life. The emotional side of her, however, finds it unacceptable. She is angry that she got this illness and none of her sisters got it. She is angry with her mother for passing on her "bad" genes. She is frustrated with psychiatrists because they can't find a cure. At a recent support group meeting, Amanda had this to say:

"It's not fair. It shouldn't have to be this way. It's not right. Why should I have to be the one that deals with this? Why should I have to take multiple medications when other people have to take only one? Why can't they find a cure? I hate taking medicines. I don't even like taking aspirin. I'm a nurse. I'm supposed to help others, not be a patient myself. This was not the way it was supposed to turn out!"

Raquel was at the same meeting and had this to offer Amanda:

"You're right that it's not fair. It's never fair that some people have to suffer more than others. And it's frustrating that scientists seem to be getting closer to a cure for so many other diseases but can't get a handle on this one. I agree that it should not be this way. You have a right to be mad. But then what do you do? I stayed mad for many years after I was diagnosed with bipolar disorder. I was even angrier when my little granddaughter was diagnosed with it. I blamed the doctors, God, and myself. I cried about it, prayed for it to go away or to be a mistake, and even tried to pretend it wasn't real. But for all my complaining and anger and tears, the spells of depression kept coming back. Staying angry didn't get me very far. Fixing the problem as best I could by following my doctor's orders gave me a chance at a new life. You have to get the big picture, Amanda. Ask yourself what you're going to do once you finish crying or being angry. Ask yourself what you can do to make tomorrow better."

• **Fact 5: Most people are not open-minded about mental illnesses or accepting of those who have one.** Amanda is a nurse, but she tells her friends that she would rather have diabetes than bipolar disorder. She would still have to take medication for the rest of her life and modify her lifestyle, but at least she wouldn't be considered "crazy." Society is slowly changing and beginning to understand that mental illnesses are illnesses like those in any other organ of the body. However, we have not evolved enough in our sophistication to fully accept people who are mentally ill. Having a mental illness may not make you any more open-minded. Even people who have bipolar disorder can be biased against other people who have mental illnesses. If you think that having a mental illness is unacceptable or is a character flaw, or that mental illnesses are not real illnesses, you will have a hard time accepting the disorder within yourself. If you can't accept that it exists, you will find it a challenge to go along with its treatment.

• **Fact 6: Most medications do not work for everyone. It is not always possible to know ahead of time whether or not a medication will work for you,** and few people find the right combination of medications on the first try. These facts can make it very hard for you to keep trying out different medications until your doctor finds one that works, because while you are trying them out you continue to experience the discomfort of symptoms. Medication changes can also be expensive, and not all health plans cover the medications your doctor might want you to try. It takes tremendous patience on your part to stick with this trial-and-error approach. In the long run it's usually worth it, but it's normal to have doubts along the way.

• **Fact 7: If you discontinue taking medications for bipolar disorder, you're at a high risk of relapsing and suffering through the consequences of becoming severely depressed or severely manic.** The common cause of relapse in bipolar disorder is going off medication. Sometimes symptoms return immediately, but other times there may be a delay. It's the delays that will give you the impression that you don't really need medication.

• **Fact 8: If you discontinue taking medications for bipolar disorder and then try to start them up again when your symptoms return, they may not be as effective.** When mood-stabilizing medications such as lithium are discontinued and then resumed at a later date, they have been found to be less effective in controlling symptoms. This has been found to be the case for antidepressant medications as well.

When Paul was a teenager, he tried to make the following argument with his doctor and his parents.

"If episodes of depression and mania occur only from time to time with periods of normal mood in between, isn't it possible that during those in-between times I don't need medication? If I went 5 years without another episode of mania, those would be 5 years I could have been off medication."

Paul would not be wrong in theory, but since recurrences of depression and mania are not always predictable and usually do not follow a uniform pattern, it's not possible to know when the next episode is coming. What is known is that without consistent medication, as a person ages the time between episodes of depression and mania will get shorter and each episode itself will tend to get longer. It took a few more experiences with severe depression before Paul was willing to concede this point.

What You Should Do If You Really Want to Take a Break from Medication

• Talk it over with your doctor. Discuss the pros and cons of doing so.
• Be certain that decreasing medications is a reasonable idea and not a manic idea. If you're uncertain, review the Mood Symptoms Worksheet that you created in Chapter 3 to determine whether you're having any symptoms of mania or depression. If so, postpone your plan until your symptoms are more stable and reevaluate.
• Ask the doctor to advise you on how to decrease the medications rather than stopping them altogether.
• Decide together how you both will know if symptoms are returning. Perhaps you can keep a Mood Graph (Chapter 4) during the transition.
• Check the Mood Symptoms Worksheet weekly to evaluate your symptoms.
• Promise yourself that you will do what is in your own best interest even if that means admitting that your plan to go off medicines did not work.
• Meet regularly with your doctor or therapist to check your progress.
• If symptoms return, meet with your doctor as soon as possible to decide how to proceed.

- Consider the possibility that even if you can manage without medications at present, it may be necessary to resume them if symptoms return.
- Be certain that going off medications is worth the risk of relapsing.

One of the most important precautions you can take is to work with your doctor to find a medication regimen that is right for you and stick with it. Most people with bipolar disorder resist the idea of taking medication at some point in their lives. So there is a good chance you have already been through this or will find it happening in the future. If you are OK with your medication now but find yourself having second thoughts about it at a later date, come back and read through this chapter. Perhaps it will help you sort through the issues.

Some clinicians think that when you do not want to take medication you are actually in denial about having bipolar disorder. While this may not always be the reason, it's a possibility.

What's Next?

It is not easy to accept a diagnosis of bipolar disorder. It is natural to seek other explanations for your symptoms and to resist the need for medication treatment. This chapter described the stages that people go through as they are trying to come to terms with the fact that they have a mental illness. Having a better understanding of your mood swings, including what makes them better and what makes them worse, can help you prepare for the future. The following chapter will help you create a plan to help control your mood swings by taking your medication more consistently.

13

Improve Medication Consistency

In this chapter you will:

✓ Set some goals for treating your mood swings.

✓ Figure out what keeps you from taking medication regularly.

✓ Use behavioral contracts to create a personal plan for treatment.

Even if you have come to terms with having bipolar disorder and agree to take medication regularly (see Chapter 12), a number of things can keep you from following the treatment regimen as prescribed by your doctor. Sometimes there are practical reasons, like running out of medication. There can be family reasons, such as your parents not accepting your diagnosis or not understanding how medications work. Medications can cause uncomfortable or dangerous side effects, and some people do not like the idea of having to take them at all. In other cases, the medications may be effective, but you may not like your doctor or the clinic where you get your prescriptions. Reliance on less effective ways to cope, like the ones described in Chapter 5, can interfere with medication treatment as can thinking errors, like the ones you read about in Chapters 7 and 10. Another common reason for not taking medications regularly is that they don't always seem to work. You can take them religiously and still have mood swings.

If you and your doctor have come to an agreement that medication treatment is called for, there are several things you can do to get the most out of it. For bipolar disorder, the most important thing is to take your medication consistently. Taking medication on a daily basis is referred to as treatment adherence. This topic has been studied a great deal because it is such a challenge to achieve. People who have to take medications for chronic health problems such as bipolar disorder, diabetes, high blood pressure, or HIV tend to be consistent for periods of time, usually when they are feeling bad. They also go through times when they take medications inconsistently or stop them altogether. This can be life threatening in some situations. Treatment adherence is hard to achieve even for short courses of medications such as antibiotics.

The goal of this chapter is to help you identify common things that can interfere with your ability to take medications consistently and create a plan to prevent or work around them. This chapter is intended for people who have decided to take medication for bipolar disorder.

Treatment Obstacles

If you have struggled with taking medications on a consistent basis, you have probably had the experience where your brain tells you to take them and you know it is a good idea, but you put it off, skip a dose, or "forget" to take them. Usually nothing bad happens right away. You may not consciously think about it, but your brain files away that information. The next time you don't want to take the pills, it is a little easier to skip a dose because you recall that nothing bad happened the last time.

This is a good example of how sometimes our thoughts and actions don't match. When that happens, you can learn a few things about yourself by observing your actions. Tommy is a good example. After returning to the hospital a second time for a manic episode that had not yet ended, Tommy agreed to take medication. At the time, he thought he understood why he needed it and thought he was convinced he should take it. But once he got home, he missed a few doses and then stopped taking the medication altogether. His mother suspected that Tommy would not really keep up with medication, so she confronted him on it and he admitted that he didn't want to take it. At first he couldn't explain why he said he would take it and then changed his mind, but when his mom handed him the bottle, he flashed on the stories from the other patients about the downside of taking medications. They talked about side effects, the expense, and never quite feeling like their usual selves again. Tommy didn't want that, and so, without consciously deciding to do so, he missed a few doses and then stopped taking medication altogether.

If you are like Tommy, you may have struggled with wanting to feel better on the one hand and not wanting to take medications on the other hand. Chapter 12 described how bargaining, a stage in coming to terms with having bipolar disorder, leads people to make deals with themselves, promising to change other habits if this will allow them to avoid having to take medication. People with chronic illnesses like type 2 diabetes or high blood pressure go through the same thing.

Exercise 13.1 on page 168 provides a list of common reasons for not taking medication consistently. If you want to do all you can to avoid the next mood swing, try to become more aware of the forces that keep you from being consistent with your medication treatment. Check off the ones you have experienced and circle the ones you need to overcome now.

In Chapter 5, you learned about coping behaviors, including some that give only

EXERCISE 13.1 Common Reasons for Not Taking
                      Medications Consistently

Listed below are common obstacles to taking medication. Check the ones that you have
experienced and circle the ones that need your immediate attention.

Practical reasons

☐ *I ran out of medicines.*

☐ *I forgot to take them.*

☐ *I don't have any money to buy my medicines.*

☐ *I don't have a ride to the pharmacy to pick up my medicines.*

Family reasons

☐ *My mom worries about my taking medicines.*

☐ *My brother had a reaction to these medicines, so I'm afraid to take them.*

☐ *My family doesn't understand why I have to take medicines.*

☐ *I need to stay alert at night so I can listen for the kids.*

Medication reasons

☐ *They make me sleepy.*

☐ *They make me gain weight.*

☐ *I don't like having to depend on medicines.*

☐ *They don't really help me.*

Doctor reasons

☐ *My doctor doesn't understand me.*

☐ *The doctor is always in a hurry and doesn't take time to listen to me.*

☐ *I don't like my doctor, the nurse, or the clinic.*

☐ *I disagree with the doctor's diagnosis.*

short-term relief. When people encounter the treatment obstacles listed in Exercise 13.1, there is a tendency to cope in ways that give immediate relief but don't really solve the problem. The best way to cope with medication obstacles is to talk with your prescribing health care provider. Work out a plan that will make you feel better, that you can tolerate well, and that fits with your lifestyle. However, most people deal with medication obstacles by ignoring or avoiding them, like Tommy does.

Amanda is a nurse, and she knows a lot about medications. In her line of work, she has seen it all—good doctors and bad ones; helpful medications and those that make symptoms worse. She does not entirely trust any doctor, including her psychiatrist, but she does trust her instincts. For these reasons, Amanda deals with her worries about medications by making small changes in her regimen from time to time. She stops and restarts them, adds "natural" treatments, alters the dose, and changes how frequently she takes them. She uses her feelings as a guide, but her feelings are affected by her mood swings.

When Amanda feels bad enough, she makes an appointment with her doctor. He lectures her on the importance of being consistent with her meds, but it goes in one ear and out the other. Amanda believes she knows what is best in spite of the fact that self-adjustment of her medications has not helped to control her symptoms. Her dislike of having to be dependent on medications and her distrust of physicians make her tinker with her medication regimen. This is a good example of how your thoughts and feelings can affect your actions in ways that can be self-defeating. However, it is ultimately Amanda's choice whether or not to follow her doctor's instructions. Working through the exercises in Chapters 7, 10, and 11 might help Amanda sort through her negative thoughts about her doctor and her treatment and perhaps come up with a better solution. She has avoided talking with her doctor about her displeasure with his care because she assumes he will not listen. Some of the ideas in Chapter 8 on coping with avoidance and procrastination might help her come up with a more effective strategy.

If you agree that taking medication consistently is a good goal, you might find it helpful to make a plan for coping with times when obstacles to treatment threaten to interfere with your good intentions. The next section will introduce behavioral contracts, a method used by therapists to help people set treatment goals and stick with them.

Plan Ahead with Behavioral Contracts

A behavioral contract is an intervention used by clinicians for helping people to set treatment goals, anticipate things that could interfere with progress and eliminate or help cope with them when they occur. Goals to address in the behavioral contract might include doing what you can to take medication regularly and as it is prescribed as well as mustering the self-discipline to use the exercises in this book or to follow the advice of your therapist or counselor. When you make a contract with yourself, you are committing to a plan that will help you gain better control over your illness.

The behavioral contract presented in Exercise 13.2A–C has three parts. In Exercise

13.2A on the facing page, you state your treatment plans. This will include your plan for taking medication, using the methods in this book, and participating in any other types of treatment you have decided to begin. These might include individual or group psychotherapy and support group meetings such as those offered by Alcoholics Anonymous (*www.aa.org*) or the Depression and Bipolar Support Alliance (*www.dbsalliance.org*).

In the second part of the behavioral contract, as shown in Exercise 13.2B (p. 172), you make a list of things that could keep you from accomplishing your goals. This will help you plan ahead for times when you might stray from your treatment goals. If you know what can interfere with your goals, you can make a plan to avoid such obstacles or to cope with them once they occur. In the third part of the behavioral contract (Exercise 13.2C on p. 172) you can make a plan to deal with each of the obstacles to treatment that you identified in the second part. You may download and print additional copies of these exercises from *www. guilford.com/basco2-forms* and add them to your workbook as needed.

Part I: Your Treatment Goals

In Part I of your personal plan for treatment, write in the medications you plan to take on a regular basis. Be specific about the dose and the times of day you want to take them. In addition to taking medications, you probably have personal goals you would like to accomplish as part of your therapy or self-help plan. Your goals might include getting yourself to stop a behavior, change a behavior, or learn something new. Sometimes your personal goals include coping better with other people. Try to be as specific as possible. For example, don't set a goal such as "being a better person." That is too general. Instead, think of a way in which you would like to change yourself. Maybe you want to stop procrastinating, get a job, control your anger, or communicate more assertively with others. These would be reasonable treatment goals.

Part II: The Obstacles

Think back to times in the past when you might have skipped medications intentionally, accidentally missed a few, run out, or decided to quit even when your doctor thought that was a bad idea. In Part II of your treatment plan, write in the factors that might have kept you from sticking with the treatment plan. Review the list of obstacles in Exercise 13.1 and write any that apply to you in Part II of the behavioral contract. Following are some questions to help you recall the factors that might have kept you from taking medications in the past as you had intended or as your doctor had recommended. Add any pertinent factors to Part II of the contract.

- What kinds of things might have influenced your decision to discontinue medication?
- Did your mood or your state of mind have anything to do with it? If so, what moods or symptoms could make you want to skip doses or stop altogether?
- Did anyone else encourage you to quit taking medicines?

EXERCISE 13.2A Your Personal Plan for Treatment, Part I: My Goals		
I intend to follow this plan for taking medication as often as possible:		
Type of medication	*Dose*	*Schedule*

My other goals for treatment include the following:

Therapy:

Self-help groups or other resources:

From *The Bipolar Workbook, Second Edition.* Copyright 2015 by The Guilford Press.

- Do you have any personal qualities or weaknesses that could have made you less consistent with treatment? How about forgetfulness, lack of organization, or impatience?
- Were you overly confident that you could handle things without medication?
- Did you have a negative attitude or just get tired of taking medication?

Part III: The Plan

Now that you know the possible pitfalls, it's time to make a plan for how you will handle each if it occurs. If you make a plan now, you will be better prepared to head off problems with medication before they interfere with your progress and recovery.

After you've created your behavioral contract, give a copy to your doctor and your therapist. Put a copy for yourself in a place where you will see it from time to time. Make it your mission to review the plan periodically.

If new situations occur that make you think about stopping your medications or at least skipping a few doses, add them to your plan, talk them over with your doctor or therapist, and try to figure out a way to keep them from interfering with your goals.

Your Personal Plan for Treatment, Part II:
The Obstacles

Use the items you marked in Exercise 13.1 to help you anticipate things that could interfere with the goals you set as part of your personal treatment plan.

It is possible that the following things could keep me from taking medication regularly:

It is possible that the following factors could keep me from participating in therapy or from using other self-help methods:

Your Personal Plan for Treatment, Part III:
The Plan

The following is my plan for overcoming the obstacles I listed in Part II:

The issue:

The plan:

The issue:

The plan:

The issue:

The plan:

Part I: My Goals

I intend to follow this plan for taking medication as often as possible:

Type of medication	Dose	Schedule
Lithium	900 mg	at night

My other goals for treatment are as follows:

Therapy: Meet with my therapist regularly for at least 6 months and work through this workbook together.

Self-help groups or other resources: I will also go to support group meetings every other month. I will make time each week to work on the exercises in this workbook.

Part II: The Obstacles

It is possible that the following factors could keep me from taking medication regularly:

Losing patience with a slow recovery

Weight gain

Getting annoyed with the doctor

It is possible that the following factors could keep me from participating in therapy or from using other self-help methods:

Being too busy to attend group meetings

Not having a quiet moment at home to work on the exercises in this book

Part III: The Plan

The following is my plan for overcoming the obstacles I listed in Part II.

The issue: Impatience.
The plan: Remember that progress takes time. Look for progress over several weeks or months rather than making decisions about medicine day by day. Stick with my plan to stay with this psychiatrist for at least 2 years.

The issue: Weight gain.
The plan: Start a weight control plan now. Start walking in the neighborhood like I used to do. Give up cookies altogether.

The issue. Annoyance with doctor.
The plan: When I get annoyed, talk to him about it like a grown-up instead of dropping out of treatment. If I have trouble doing it, I can ask my therapist to help.

The issue: Too busy.
The plan: Make time to help myself. Make myself a higher priority than I have in the past. If I can make time to vacuum, I can make time to work on myself.

The issue: No quiet time.
The plan: I can find time when I want to. I can go to work a half hour early and sit in the cafeteria where it is quiet, or I can take time on Saturday morning before the kids wake up.

Find a time to regularly review your goals. Amanda has decided that she will review the plan before each appointment with her psychiatrist. Raquel has been on the same medication regimen for years and has no trouble sticking with it. She reviews her plan when she sees her doctor, every 6 months. Paul has his plan on his computer as a screen saver. It pops up from time to time to remind him of his goals. He updates it regularly. Tommy is not quite ready to make a behavioral contract. He needs time to work on his acceptance of the illness before he is willing to make a long-term commitment to treatment. He skipped over Chapter 12, but he is going to go back and read it. When he is ready, he will give the contract idea some thought.

The sections that follow offer some suggestions for common problems with taking medications regularly. Pick the solutions that suit you best or modify these suggestions to fit your own situation. Write your ideas for coping with these situations in Part III of your behavioral contract.

Common Problems with Taking Medications

There are some concerns about taking medications that are common for many people with bipolar disorder. In fact, taking medications consistently for long periods of time is a problem for most people with chronic illnesses. Several examples are presented in the sections below along with some suggestions for dealing with these problems.

"I sometimes forget to take my medication. What should I do?"

• **Suggestion 1:** Always take your medicine at the same time each day. Make it a routine, just like putting on your shoes each day or brushing your teeth.

• **Suggestion 2:** Use a divided pillbox for your medication. Check the box midday to be sure you've taken your medication. Put the box in a place where you are likely to see it each day. If you see it, you'll be more likely to take your medication.

• **Suggestion 3:** Write a note to yourself that reminds you to take your medication. Put the note in a place where you will see it each day. Some common places to put reminder notes include your refrigerator, near your bathroom mirror, or in your car.

• **Suggestion 4:** Most people have a daily routine or set of daily habits. Some examples of daily routine or habits include:

  • Getting up at the same time each day
  • Brushing your teeth in the morning
  • Drinking your morning coffee
  • Getting dressed for the day
  • Watching certain television shows

• A way to remember to take your medications regularly is to take them at the same time that you complete one of your other daily routines or habits. For example, you might take your medicine with your morning coffee.

"I don't think I need these medicines anymore. What should I do?"

• **Suggestion 1:** Before you decide to stop taking your medication, talk with your doctor about your concerns. Some medications should be taken daily even when you're feeling better. The purpose of these medications is to keep your symptoms from returning. If you're feeling fine now, it's probably because the medication is working well.

• **Suggestion 2:** Having the urge to stop taking medications and feeling like you don't need them anymore might really be a sign that the illness is getting worse. To be certain, before stopping any medications, talk with your doctor. Be sure you are making a good decision. The desire to stop taking medication is sometimes a signal that the symptoms are returning or are getting worse.

If you are depressed, it can feel like the medication is not helping, like nothing can help. Sometimes people feel hopeless or overwhelmed and don't know what to do. They may end up thinking it would be better to stop taking their medication.

This way of thinking is actually a sign that depression is getting worse. It would not be the best time to stop taking medication, but it would be a good time to see your doctor and ask for help.

If you are getting manic, you might feel really good, better than usual, and think you don't need medication anymore. This is called hypomania. It is the early stage of mania. Hypomania can very quickly turn into mania, especially if you stop taking your medications. Before you make the decision to stop your medicines, ask someone else for an opinion on how you are doing.

"Some of my family members don't think I should take medication. What should I do?"

When family members discourage you from taking medications, it's usually because they have worries or concerns about them. Sometimes people have heard stories about medications that scared them. In trying to protect you from harm, they might tell you not to take them or question your need for them.

The usual problem is that family members may not understand your illness or the purpose of taking medications. They might need more information or education from your doctor or therapist.

Here are some ways to get them the information they need.

• **Suggestion 1:** Ask one of your family members to come with you to your next doctor's appointment. If only one family member can come to your appointment, choose one who can talk with the other members of your family and share what is learned during the visit.

Tell your doctor that the family is worried about your taking medications. The doctor will help your family understand more about your illness and will explain the purpose of the medications. Your family members will have an opportunity to ask questions about their concerns or fears.

- **Suggestion 2:** Ask your doctor for some written information about your illness and its treatment. Give this information to your family members.

- **Suggestion 3:** Invite your family members to go with you to a support group meeting such as one held by the Depression and Bipolar Support Alliance (DBSA) or the National Alliance on Mental Illness (NAMI). These groups provide information for family members about mental illnesses and their treatments.

- **Suggestion 4:** Thank your family members for their concern. Tell them where they can get more information about your treatment. Let them know that you have decided to take the medication to control your symptoms.

"I don't like the way my medication makes me feel."

Side effects are one of the most common reasons that people stop taking their medications. For many medications, however, the side effects are temporary. They occur when you first begin taking medication or when you change your dose. If you miss taking your medication for a few days and start up again, your side effects may return. Sometimes side effects from medication can persist even after you've been taking medication for some time.

- **Suggestion 1:** Talk to your doctor about the way your medications make you feel. Ask whether the discomforts are a result of medication or a separate problem altogether. If you're experiencing side effects, ask your doctor how long they are likely to last and whether anything can be done about it. Follow the doctor's advice. If you give it enough time and still feel uncomfortable, talk with your doctor again.

- **Suggestion 2:** Because doctors are more familiar with the side effects of medication than you are, they may not be as concerned as you when they occur. They may assess your problem and tell you the symptoms will pass. If you sense a lack of concern or feel that your doctor has dismissed your complaints too quickly, calmly tell the doctor what you are thinking. Ask why he or she does not seem worried. Make sure you've made it clear just how bothersome the side effects are.

- **Suggestion 3:** If the side effects are not likely to go away, consider whether the benefits you get from the medication may be worth tolerating the side effects. If the medication keeps you from getting depressed or manic, maybe it's worth tolerating the annoying side effects. When you're feeling well, it's easy to focus on the side effect as being the biggest annoyance in your life. When you were having severe symptoms, you felt so bad that the side effects may not have mattered. Think it through before you stop your medication.

"I'm afraid to take medications."

It's normal to feel afraid of new treatments. You may wonder if you've received the right diagnosis and whether the medications you were prescribed are really the best choices for you. If you've heard stories about bad experiences people have had when taking medication, you might be concerned that you could have a bad experience also.

• **Suggestion 1:** Ask your doctor plenty of questions about the medicine. Start by asking some of the following:

> • "Why did you choose these particular medications for me?"
> • "Could there be any bad side effects? If so, what are they?"
> • "What should I do if I start to feel the side effects?"
> • "Whom should I call? Should I stop them right away?"

• **Suggestion 2:** Talk to other people who have taken the same medication and have done all right. Ask them about the things that worry you.

If any of the situations previously described apply to you, you might be able to add some of the coping suggestions to Part III of your behavioral contract. To help you get started, Amanda's completed behavioral contract is provided as an example. Amanda has had difficulty being consistent with her medications for many years. She wants to have a more stable life and is eager to do her part to make that happen. She has struggled with acceptance of the illness but feels that she has turned the corner and is ready to deal with it.

What's Next?

Mood swings caused by bipolar disorder generally require medication treatment to control them. Although there are many strategies in this book to help you manage your symptoms, the underlying illness that creates the mood swings requires a medical intervention to prevent mood swings into depression and mania from recurring. For the medication to be most effective, you have to take it as prescribed. Skipping doses or stopping and starting medications can compromise their effectiveness. The goal of this chapter was helping you prepare to cope with common obstacles to taking medication consistently as well as obstacles that can interfere with other aspects of your treatment. You can adjust the plan as your treatment changes or as you eliminate or identify new obstacles to treatment. In the next chapter you will learn how to strengthen your problem-solving skills. If you had trouble completing the third part of your personal plan for treatment, apply the skills in Chapter 14 to the obstacles that still need solutions.

Strengthen Your Coping Skills

14

Effectively Solve Problems

In this chapter you will:

- ✓ Learn the four steps to effective problem solving.

- ✓ Discover the importance of clearly defining problems.

- ✓ Develop strategies for picking the best solution.

- ✓ Pick up tips on how to solve problems that involve other people.

A Step-by-Step Approach to Solving Problems

People start learning to be problem solvers when they are babies. The problems that need attention early in life are simple compared to ones faced in adulthood, but the skills needed are very similar. It starts with becoming aware of a problem, analyzing it, and reasoning through and/or trying out solutions until the problem is solved. If no solution is found, we adapt. It is all very systematic.

It is much harder to solve problems when you are exhausted, depressed, overwhelmed, or can't concentrate. Mood swings can make you forget that you possess problem-solving skills. Instead, when you are faced with difficulties, instinctual coping behaviors kick in, like the ones described in Chapter 5. The goal of this workbook is to help you make use of and strengthen your coping skills, or to develop new ones. This chapter focuses on strengthening your problem-solving skills. It takes you back to the basics of defining a problem, identifying possible solutions, and creating a plan of action.

Define the Problem

The most difficult part of solving problems is clearly describing the nature of the problem. While difficult, it's an essential step. If you can clearly see the problem, you can solve it or cope with it. Using vague or general terms that do not fully describe what is happening will not lead you to a solution. Some examples of vague and clear definitions of problems are provided in Exercise 14.1 below. Notice that the problems as stated in the left column could mean many different things. The definitions in the right column are stated more clearly and give you a better idea of what the person really intended to say. As you read through each unclear problem, try to think of what the statement means to you. Practice by adding specific language to each one to clarify how you would define each problem.

Your definition of the problem should point you toward its solution. In the examples in the table, Paul needs to clean his apartment, and Raquel needs to find money to pay the phone bill, ask the phone company to give her a break, or deal with having her phone service stopped. Tommy needs to make a decision to talk to his friends about being left out of the party or to get over it if it's not important enough to discuss with them. Amanda needs to find out if she will be fired soon and whether or not there is anything that can be done to stop it. If she is not sure what to do next, it may be time to begin looking for other job options or to ask others for advice or assistance.

To help you define and describe a problem clearly enough to solve it, ask yourself the questions in Exercise 14.2 on page 183. You may download and print additional copies of this exercise from *www.guilford.com/basco2-forms* and add them to your workbook as needed.

Now that you have a better idea of the nature of your problem, you are ready to describe it in enough detail to help you begin to generate solutions. Exercise 14.3 (p. 183) provides a

---

EXERCISE 14.1   Clear and Unclear Definitions of Problems

Compare the clear and unclear definitions of common problems provided below. Try to figure out what's wrong with the way the problems in the left column are stated. How might you state the problem if it was happening to you?

Unclear definitions	Examples of clearer definitions
Paul thinks, "*I'm lazy.*"	*I have not cleaned the apartment in several weeks.*
Raquel says, "*I'm broke.*"	*I may not have enough money to pay my phone bill this month because I had to get my car fixed.*
Tommy thinks, "*No one cares about me.*"	*My friends had a get-together this weekend, and no one invited me.*
Amanda says, "*I'm going to lose it if I get fired for doing the right thing.*"	*It's possible that I will lose my job for walking off before the end of my shift. I'm not sure if I will be able to find another job this time.*

EXERCISE 14.2 Ten Questions to Define a Problem

Pick a problem that is currently bothering you. Use the following questions to hone in on a clear definition of the problem.

1. What is the problem?

2. Is it something that happened in the past or something that still needs to be resolved?

3. Is it your problem or someone else's problem?

4. Is there anything you can do about it right now?

5. When is it most likely to occur?

6. How often does the problem occur?

7. If it does not get solved, what will happen?

8. What is your biggest worry about this problem?

9. If it were solved, how would things be different for you?

10. What part of the problem needs to be solved first?

From *The Bipolar Workbook, Second Edition.* Copyright 2015 by The Guilford Press.

EXERCISE 14.3 Summarize the Problem

Based on your answers to the questions in Exercise 14.2, try to clearly define your problem in Exercise 14.3.

The problem is:

The way it affects my life is:

It upsets me because:

It has to be resolved soon because:

From *The Bipolar Workbook, Second Edition.* Copyright 2015 by The Guilford Press.

PAUL'S EXAMPLE   Summarize the Problem

The problem is: *that my apartment is a mess.*

The way it affects my life is: *that it distracts me and makes me feel bad.*

It upsets me because: *I hate living in a disaster area.*

It has to be resolved soon because: *people might be coming over this weekend.*

RAQUEL'S EXAMPLE   Summarize the Problem

The problem is: *I don't have enough money.*

The way it affects my life is: *that I can't pay all my bills.*

It upsets me because: *this keeps happening to us. I hate living like this.*

It has to be resolved soon because: *the bills are coming due.*

TOMMY'S EXAMPLE   Summarize the Problem

The problem is: *my friends blew me off.*

The way it affects my life is: *I had nothing to do that night and I don't know why they did this.*

It upsets me because: *these people are supposed to be my friends. I have lost friends before because of the problems I have had. I don't want to lose these.*

It has to be resolved soon because: *it is going to keep bothering me until I know what happened.*

structure for clearly defining a problem. Try to be specific about why it is troublesome and why it is important to fix at this time. Taking the idea out of your head and putting it on paper is a good way to be sure that you are clear in your own mind about what needs to be fixed. After you have completed Exercise 14.3, cross-check your clarity by telling another person what is bothering you and asking if he or she understands. You may download and print additional copies of this exercise from *www.guilford.com/basco2-forms* and add them to your workbook as needed.

Find Solutions

The next step in problem solving is to put together a list of possible solutions. You can use Exercise 14.4 below to list your ideas. Try to come up with at least five possible solutions. One solution might be to change nothing and let the problem continue. Another might be to ask someone to solve it for you. While these may not be the best solutions, at least they are possibilities. Let yourself be as creative as possible in generating new solutions to your problem. Do not stop to evaluate each one as you think of it. Just make a list first and follow the steps

EXERCISE 14.4	Possible Solutions to My Problem
Order	**Ideas**

From *The Bipolar Workbook, Second Edition.* Copyright 2015 by The Guilford Press.

AMANDA'S EXAMPLE	Possible Solutions to My Problem
Order	**Ideas**
	Apologize to my boss for walking out before the end of my shift.
	Keep my mouth shut and wait to see what happens.
	Start looking for another job. Quit before I get fired.
	Ask my boss if she plans to fire me because I walked out without an explanation.
	Ask the unit secretary if she knows anything about her plan to fire me.

for choosing the right one. You may download and print additional copies of this exercise from *www.guilford.com/basco2-forms* and add them to your workbook as needed.

After you have filled in at least five possible solutions, cross off the ones that are least desirable or not very practical given your current situation. Think about the pros and cons of each of the remaining solutions and put them in order of preference. In the column on the left labeled "Order," write "1" next to your first choice, "2" next to your second choice, and so on. Solution 1 will usually be the first one you will try. If it looks like it's not going to work, go to solution 2 and so on.

Amanda has been fired twice for walking off a job in anger, and she does not want it to happen again. She knows she will be better off quitting before getting fired, but she doesn't want to jump the gun. She likes her job and the pay is good, so she would really rather not lose it. It would be better for her in the long run to do what she can to try to keep her job.

Amanda knows in her heart that she should probably apologize for getting irritated and walking off the unit before her shift ended, but that's not easy for her to do. She is a proud woman and believes that it was best to walk away rather than take out her irritability on the staff or on a patient. Her shift was nearly over and no one was in crisis at the time. She doesn't know how to apologize, especially because she thinks she made the right call.

She could also just ask her boss directly about her plans to fire her without apologizing. If it looked like she was heading in that direction, she could offer to resign instead. The problem with that idea is that she doesn't want to resign and she would not get unemployment benefits if she resigned.

Amanda thought the wait-and-see method sounded like the easiest. She knew that sometimes she blew things out of proportion and jumped to conclusions about getting fired, so this could be another example of overreaction. Maybe her boss understood why Amanda left a little early and would agree that it was the best thing to do. Maybe there was no problem. However, after thinking it over, Amanda decided the best strategy would be to apologize to her boss and explain what happened. Even if she was not about to fire her, offering an explanation and an apology was probably the right thing to do. If Amanda was going to get fired, she would find out soon enough and would still have the option of offering to resign. It would be better for her and better for the hospital.

Refine Your Plan

Before you put your plan into action, give some thought to when you will try it. Is the solution something you need to do right away, or do you need more time to prepare before you act on it? If you have been avoiding the problem, it may be helpful to make a commitment to yourself to fix it by picking a specific day and time to implement your plan. To increase the chance that you will follow through, put the date on your calendar and tell someone else about your plan.

Some plans require assistance or cooperation from other people. Will you need help and, if so, what kind of help? Do you need practical assistance, transportation, moral support, or some other kind of help? Think about who might be able to help you and tell them about the day and time you are planning to get started. You may have to make adjustments depending on their schedule. Plan ahead. Do not wait until the last minute to ask for help.

Sometimes the solution to a problem requires the cooperation of others, especially if your problem involves them. For example, you may have created a plan for getting to work on time, but the solution involves getting someone else to wake you in the morning. You will need the cooperation of that person to make the plan work. If other people are involved, talk over your ideas with them, get their suggestions, and make an agreement on when each of you will take action.

A good plan is one that works. Before you take action, figure out what outcome you expect. How will you know if your plan worked? If it is something straightforward like getting to work on time, your clock at work will tell you if you succeeded. If you are trying to achieve something more complex, such as improving your self-esteem, a good outcome may be more difficult to detect. Give some thought to the outcome you would achieve if you were able to improve your self-esteem. Maybe you are looking for a change in yourself like less self-criticism about your appearance. Be sure to choose an outcome that is within your control. For example, if your goal is to improve your self-esteem, do not use attention from other people as your indicator of success. You have no control over other people's behavior. Exercise 14.5 below will help you put the final touches on your plan. You may download and print additional copies of this exercise from *www.guilford.com/basco2-forms* and add them to your workbook as needed.

Put Your Plan into Action

The next step is to try out your solution and see what happens. If the solution does not seem to work at first, make a decision to try it again or switch to solution 2 from your list.

EXERCISE 14.5 Refine Your Plan

Firm up your plan by adding details about the timing, the people involved, and the outcome.

When?

Who will help?

How will you know if the plan worked?

> **AMANDA'S EXAMPLE** **Refine Your Plan**
>
> **When?** *I will practice my apology tonight with my husband and talk to my boss tomorrow at work. If she emails me or calls me tonight, I will apologize right away.*
>
> **Who will help?** *My husband will help me figure out what to say. I will ask a friend at work to give me some feedback on how she thinks the boss will react.*
>
> **How will you know if the plan worked?** *If my apology works, she will give me a warning and not fire me.*

Sometimes you have to try the same solution more than once before it will work. If Amanda's apology note does not seem to make a difference, she may need to try again in person.

In other situations you may find that your first solution was not sufficient to address a problem. If that's the case, try another solution from your list.

If Amanda is uncertain about how her apology was received, she might ask the unit's secretary about it. Although she wishes she could just wait and see what happens to her job, Amanda knows that the wait will make her feel worse. If her first solution, the apology, does not work, she will ask her boss if she plans to fire her for walking out without an explanation.

Learn from your experiences of success as well as failure. As you get to know yourself better—your motivations, your weaknesses, your abilities, and your needs—you will be able to choose solutions that best suit you.

People Problems

The skills you learned in Chapter 11 for sorting out thoughts, feelings, and actions can be used in conjunction with the skills in this chapter to address problems that involve other people. Events with others trigger an emotional reaction in both people. Those reactions can cause new problems. To set things right, you sometimes have to sort through the negative thoughts until you can identify the real problem. Then you can use the problem-solving steps in this chapter to try to resolve things.

Actions and Reactions

Joe provides a good example of this. Joe has been married to Sarah for nearly 20 years and has struggled with bipolar II disorder and periodic drinking problems for the past 15 years. He has lost jobs due to periods of severe depression but has worked his way up to a management position and has been sober for 3 years. Joe has been putting in a lot of overtime hours on his new job at the store and has been exhausted and unable to do much once he gets home from work. Sarah has been highly supportive and glad to see Joe doing so well and enjoying his work, although she has been somewhat concerned that his extra energy may be a sign of hypomania. The following example illustrates Joe's and Sarah's reactions to Joe's getting a raise. Take notice of how their differing feelings and thoughts created a problem for them and how they solved it. To help us examine their problem more closely, it is broken down into two parts or events.

Event 1: Joe gets a raise		
Joe's feelings	**Joe's thoughts**	**Joe's actions**
Joy, excitement	*This is terrific. I've been working hard. I deserve a reward.*	Joe stopped off at the local casino on the way home, had a few drinks, spent a little too much money, and got into an argument with his wife when he got home.
Sarah's feelings	**Sarah's thoughts**	**Sarah's actions**
Pride, relief from worries about money, happy for Joe	*This is terrific. Now we can get a better handle on our credit card bills.*	Sarah wrote and mailed a check to the credit card company for more than the minimum payment. Later she got angry with Joe and yelled at him when he came home from the casino smelling like alcohol.

Event 2: Joe's wife yells at him		
Joe's feelings	**Joe's thoughts**	**Joe's actions**
Angry, upset with his wife for yelling at him	*I can't do anything right for that woman. She does not appreciate how hard I work. She doesn't trust me. I don't have to take this.*	Joe left the house, went to a neighborhood bar, and had a few more drinks. He woke up late for work the next day and was reprimanded by his boss. He felt awful.
Sarah's feelings	**Sarah's thoughts**	**Sarah's actions**
Angry, sad, and discouraged	*Here we go again with the drinking. Just when things seemed to be going our way, Joe messes up everything. I can't take this anymore.*	Sarah canceled the check to the credit card company. She ignored Joe for several days, then later criticized him for not helping out enough at home. Her anger stayed with her for several days.

This is a typical example of how reactions to events can lead to new problems and can extend a mild mood swing into a major mood episode in people who have an underlying mood disorder. Joe might have had a mild case of hypomania that was giving him more energy and excitement on the job. It made him perform well, but it also may have impaired his judgment. He made matters worse by his choice of actions after hearing that he got a raise—after calling Sarah with the good news he celebrated at the local casino, drank alcohol after 3 years of sobriety, and gambled money that he could not afford to spend. To get himself out of the situation, Joe needed to use his resources—support from his family and AA sponsor—and take positive action by apologizing to his wife, discontinuing his drinking, and resuming his good work ethic. Once his mood was back to normal, he needed to stay vigilant about his mood symptoms and be mindful of the warning signs of another significant mood episode.

Sarah has been through a lot in helping Joe cope with his mood swings and his addiction. She enjoyed his last 3 years of sobriety and thought his problems were behind them. Joe's recent setback triggered a lot of distress for Sarah, negatively affecting her concentration at work, her patience with the kids, and her interactions with Joe. Sarah does not have a mood disorder, so her mood improved and she was able to let go of the event as soon as Joe showed signs of improvement.

Sarah and Joe had been to counseling in the past. They had both learned how their moods were affected by stressful events. They both learned that their choices of action could either make things better or make things worse. Their marital therapist had trained them to stop and look at their reactions to stressful events and to change directions if they seemed to be going down a destructive path. They did this by asking themselves four questions that they learned from their therapist:

1. "WHAT WERE YOU THINKING?"

- Joe thought of his trip to the casino as a reward for his hard work.
- Sarah saw it as Joe breaking a promise not to drink and as irresponsible given that they could not afford to waste money on gambling.

2. "WHY DID YOU DO THAT?"

- Joe went to the casino and had a few drinks to reward himself. After Sarah yelled at him, he went to a bar because he was angry with her, he didn't want to deal with her, and he wanted to make the point that he could do as he pleased.
- Sarah yelled at him because she was angry.

3. "HOW DID IT MAKE YOU FEEL?"

- Drinking made Joe feel good in the short run and bad in the long run.
- Yelling at Joe made Sarah feel better in the short run, but she regretted it in the long run because it escalated their problems.

4. "IF YOU COULD DO IT ALL AGAIN, WHAT WOULD YOU DO DIFFERENTLY?"

- Joe would have gone home and celebrated his good news with his family.
- Sarah would have tried to express herself in a way that would not have escalated the situation.

Positive and negative changes in your mood and thought processes can color the types of actions you choose to take, such as staying out late to have fun because you feel terrific and don't want the day to end, yelling at others to vent your anger, or avoiding interactions with others because you're feeling bad about yourself and don't want others to see you depressed. If you can learn to recognize your thoughts and your mood before you take action, you can make better choices and avoid or reduce a negative mood swing. Asking yourself questions like the ones learned by Joe and Sarah can help you to learn from your experiences so that you can choose a different way to cope the next time.

There will be times when the solutions that Joe and Sarah generated will come in handy. They know that marriage is not easy and that problems can return. They also know that Joe's bipolar disorder will always be there and that his mood swings can affect their marriage. Working through exercises together for problems that affect them both is another way to use this workbook.

Dealing with Difficult People

The world is full of difficult people and complicated situations. You may always try to do the right thing and say the right thing but still find that you are in a no-win situation. People with severe mood swings often face the challenge of having to deal with difficult people when they are not feeling at their best. In those situations you are more likely to rely on the instinctual coping behaviors described in Chapters 5 and 8 and react from emotion rather than from logic. So what can you do about it?

DIFFICULT PEOPLE CAN TRIGGER MOOD SWINGS

It is a common misconception among psychotherapy buffs that people can't make you feel bad, only you can make yourself feel bad. This isn't true. The words and behavior of others can hurt and offend you, make you feel sad or angry, and bring out the worst in you. It is normal for humans to react negatively when presented with negative situations and people. You learned about triggers in Chapter 5 and how your natural coping instincts can sometimes make matters worse. The offensive behavior of others is a common trigger, even for people who do not have bipolar disorder.

The problem-solving steps described earlier in this chapter can help when you have to cope with difficult people. Pick a recurring situation with a difficult person (a cranky boss) that repeatedly makes you feel bad or focus on a single event (a divorce) involving another person whose effects have continued to linger. Use the questions in Exercise 14.2 to figure out what it is about the situation that troubles you most. Put some thought into the outcome you would like to achieve through problem solving. Keep in mind that you will probably not be able to change the other person unless he or she sees some value in making a change. You can, however, change how you handle upsetting situations. You will still have an initial negative reaction when difficult people behave badly—that's normal. But you can learn to analyze your reactions, correct any distortions in your thinking, and find a solution that prevents painful events from continuing to take their toll on you.

DON'T LET DIFFICULT PEOPLE MAKE YOU LOSE YOUR GAINS

Beginning with Chapter 5, you have been reading about and learning skills for controlling your mood swings. By now you have an idea of what constitute good coping behaviors and poor coping behaviors—those that give only temporary relief, do not solve the problem, or make you feel worse. Interactions with difficult people can be so overwhelming that you can forget to use your new coping skills; you revert to your old coping behaviors instead. It will take some discipline to learn to step back from uncomfortable situations and look at them objectively. Being objective will help you be a good problem solver.

Use the exercises in this workbook to make notes on how you would like to be able to handle upsetting events and people. Keep the workbook handy and review your work from time to time. Use it as a visual cue to remind you that you have skills for controlling mood swings. You do not have to rely on dysfunctional coping strategies. You can learn to cope better to feel better.

DIFFICULT PEOPLE CAN MAKE YOU DOUBT YOURSELF

When Raquel and her husband were still married, he sometimes said hurtful things to her that would leave her sobbing. He criticized her appearance, her intelligence, her cooking, her family, and her beliefs. Because she loved him and trusted him, she heard his criticisms as truth. His words would crush her, bring her to her knees in sorrow, and make her want to die. He was so convincing that she bought into it, and it took many years and a lot of therapy to bring back her self-esteem.

Raquel's husband ultimately solved her problem by leaving her while she was in the hospital for a suicide attempt. She didn't see it as a solution right away because she was convinced that she was worthless and no one would want her. Raquel's friends thought she just needed to meet a nice man who would convince her of her worth, but they were wrong. Raquel's new problem was that even though her husband was gone, his hurtful words were still in her head.

Raquel used Exercises 14.1 and 14.2 to help her define her problems. This was not an easy task. She had to seek help from a therapist to figure out what was wrong with her. She had been trying to fix the weaknesses her husband saw in her without considering the possibility that he had been wrong the whole time. The following (p. 193) is what she concluded.

Once Raquel was able to clearly define the problem, she was able to develop skills to solve it. She used the exercises in Chapters 10 and 11 to help her change her negative outlook on herself and her life.

RAQUEL'S EXAMPLE Summarize the Problem

The problem is: *that I think very little of myself. I let my husband tear down my self-worth. I see myself through his eyes.*

The way it affects my life is: *that I avoid starting new relationships. I don't think I'm good enough for anyone.*

It upsets me because: *I'm lonely. I feel like I can't change. I'm also angry with myself that I allowed him to hurt me so much. I'm stupid.*

It has to be resolved soon because: *I still have thoughts of suicide from time to time. I need to get over him.*

What's Next?

The goal of this chapter was to reintroduce you to basic problem-solving skills. By making the process more systematic, you can move from distress to problem identification and resolution. The biggest challenge is to clearly identify the nature of the problem and what you hope to gain by its resolution. Once you can see the problem, you can begin to solve it. The next chapter will help you strengthen your ability to manage stress and develop other healthy habits.

15

Strengthen Stress Management Skills and Healthy Habits

In this chapter you will:

✓ Learn how to strengthen your coping skills.

✓ Identify resources that can help you cope with stress and mood symptoms.

✓ Learn how to ask for help.

The previous chapters have focused on identifying symptoms of mood swings and using the strategies described to reduce the symptoms. You learned to monitor changes in your mood so that you can intervene as quickly as possible to keep symptoms from worsening. This chapter is a little different. The emphasis in the sections that follow is on prevention. Managing stress and developing healthy habits are two strategies for reducing the risk of mood swings, even those that are part of bipolar disorder.

All of the strategies you learned to correct negative thinking and take action can be used to deal with day-to-day stress. You don't have to wait for a major mood swing to use them. There are additional things you can do to manage your stress. They involve developing or strengthening healthy habits and keeping your stress low enough to manage. As you work through the following exercises, think about how they can help you even when you are not in a depressive, hypomanic, or manic episode.

Add Healthy Habits

In Exercise 15.1 below, list the healthy habits you already have and those you would like to develop or strengthen. Include better ways to manage your symptoms, organize your life, and get more enjoyment out of life.

EXERCISE 15.1   Healthy Habits

Healthy habits I practice regularly:

Healthy habits I need to strengthen:

New healthy habits I would like to develop:

Healthy habits I used to have and would like to restart:

TOMMY'S EXAMPLE   Healthy Habits

Healthy habits I practice regularly:
I exercise pretty often.
I avoid eating French fries and chips.

Healthy habits I need to strengthen:
Getting up on time for school
Getting to bed sooner

New healthy habits I would like to develop:
Read more
Drink alcohol less often
Stop getting speeding tickets

Healthy habits I used to have and would like to restart:
Eat healthily
Get all my homework done
Go to every class

Weight Control

Weight gain is one of the more common complaints of people who take medications for bipolar disorder. Not all the blame can be placed on medications, however. It's easy to develop poor eating habits and to put off regular exercise. Medications may make you crave unhealthy foods, and depression can make you seek out pleasure from food. But once you start eating high-fat or high-sugar foods and neglecting the healthier options, it's easy to get hooked on them. Some people try to justify their bad eating habits by saying that since they have to suffer with bipolar disorder, they have the right to enjoy the foods they like. Others say that eating is the only pleasure they have in life. Neither of these ideas would be so bad if comfort foods didn't make you gain weight.

It may be a good idea to diet and exercise, but many people put it off. When told by their doctors to start a diet program or exercise plan, they might initially resist, raising objections like those listed in Exercise 15.2 below. Circle the ones that apply to you.

It's true that changing your eating habits can be a big challenge and exercise can be hard to do. But most people want to get in better shape so that they can do more and feel better about themselves. If you follow the logic that it's easier to add a positive than take away a negative, you can make positive changes to your eating habits and activity that might help you control your weight. Start with one positive habit until you have mastered it and then add another. When you feel more confident that you can make changes, start eliminating negatives. Exercise 15.3 on the facing page lists some examples of positives you can add that will help you work toward healthier dietary and activity habits. As you read through the list, think about the ones you might be able to do.

If you think improving your eating habits and exercise is more than you can handle, go back to Chapter 9 on feeling overwhelmed and use the exercise for breaking down the task before taking it on. It will help you figure out where to start.

Once you've added some healthy habits, you may be ready to eliminate a few unhealthy ones. Exercise 15.4 on the facing page contains a list of negative habits you might consider eliminating. Try to make a change in one and master it before adding another.

EXERCISE 15.2 Weight Control Obstacles

- "I don't know how to diet."
- "I hate to exercise."
- "I can't handle a diet right now."
- "I don't want to diet."
- "It will stress me out too much."

- "I don't have money for diet foods."
- "I can't afford a gym membership."
- "It shouldn't matter that I'm fat."
- "I've tried and can't do it."
- "I like sweets."

EXERCISE 15.3 Add These Positives to Control Weight and Get Fit

- Read a book on dieting
- Join Weight Watchers
- Read the nutritional labels on foods
- Choose items that are healthier for you
- Add a piece of fruit to your lunch
- Find a vegetable that you like to eat
- Cook meals more often

- Go for a walk every day
- Scrub floors, mow the lawn, rake leaves
- Watch an exercise show on TV and try to follow along
- Walk your dog farther than usual
- Wear a pedometer
- Play with a young child

It's easy to think of diet programs in an all-or-nothing way: You either have to do it all—make all the positive changes, deny yourself "bad" foods, eat on a consistent schedule, totally work the program—or not do it at all. Coping with bipolar disorder is hard enough. Trying to follow a diet program 100% of the time may get you the best results, but if it's too difficult, you won't stick with it. Exercise 15.5 on the next page includes some general ideas that may help you improve your eating habits.

EXERCISE 15.4 Eliminating Negatives to Control Weight and Get Fit

Put a check next to the ones that might be right for you.

- Do not keep junk food at home. If you want a treat, go out and buy one serving. If it is at your fingertips, it will be harder to resist.

- Look through your grocery cart before you check out. Count how many items you are about to buy that would be considered unhealthy. If there are several, take some out. The clerk will be happy to reshelve them for you.

- Try to go without sweets for a few days until your cravings decrease.

- Trade out full-sugar soft drinks for diet drinks or water.

- Try to eat a meal without adding bread.

- Eat grilled instead of fried foods.

- Count how many sweets you eat in a day and challenge yourself to reduce them by half.

EXERCISE 15.5   Ways to Improve Your Eating Habits

Put a check next to the ones you already do and two checks next to the ones you want to try.

- Think before you eat. Make choices that are better for you.

- Use your resources. You don't have to do this alone. Ask for help.

- Join a group of people who are working toward the same goal.

- Do the best you can as often as you can rather than approaching it in an all-or-nothing way.

- Set a series of small personal goals instead of a large weight-loss goal.

- Remember that one meal or one day of poor eating does not blow the whole plan. Just make a commitment to yourself to do better the next day.

- Weight loss takes time. Don't expect overnight changes and then feel discouraged if change doesn't come right away.

- Before you buy foods labeled *low-fat*, read the label and compare the calorie count and carbohydrate content to those of the regular version.

- Ask yourself how hungry you really are before you eat. If you're just bored and not hungry, do something else. If you're upset and not really hungry at all, use one of the other methods in this workbook to help you feel better. If you're just thirsty, drink something and reevaluate your hunger afterward. If you *are* hungry, eat an amount that matches the amount of hunger you feel. Sometimes a small amount of food will do the trick. Remember, you can save the rest for later.

Relaxation Exercises to Reduce Tension

Over the years, you've probably been told to "just relax" when you worry or are stressed. If you are like many others, you undoubtedly find that advice irritating, because you know that it is easier said than done. The ability to relax is a coping skill that can help you manage stress. It comes naturally to some, but those who have mood swings usually have to work hard at it. Working hard may seem like the opposite of relaxation, but when mood symptoms affect your thoughts, feelings, and actions, you can't just "chill out" on command. You have to use your coping resources to reduce anxiety, tension, and stress.

When you make it a point to use the coping resources you listed in Chapter 5, you probably feel more relaxed. Similarly, if you try the methods in Chapter 9 you will likely feel less overwhelmed and therefore less tense. If the skills in Chapter 8 helped you stop avoiding and procrastinating, you may also have experienced the added benefit of feeling relieved. Relaxation can also occur when you reduce your negative thoughts with the methods in Chapter 9 and when you solve problems like you learned to do in Chapter 14. In each of these chapters, you began learning to change your emotions from high stress to low stress by either changing your actions or your thoughts. Sometimes, however, you need a more direct approach.

When you think stressful thoughts, your body responds by tensing and preparing you to confront the problem. If you don't take action or change your point of view, you can stay in a state of continued tension. When your body relaxes, that tension diminishes. You experience this when you sleep—the ultimate state of relaxation. If you can learn to relax the tension in your body while awake, you will find that it has a positive effect on your thoughts and feelings. For example, if you have ever sat in a comfortable chair looking out at a beautiful sunset, you may recall that your problems and worries faded away even if just for a short while. You felt at peace. Physical relaxation can reduce mental tension. There are many ways to physically relax, such as lying on a sofa watching television, taking a warm bath, or even walking in a quiet, peaceful place. The tension in your body diminishes and your mood improves.

In Exercise 15.6 on page 200, you will learn a method for reducing muscular tension in your body as a way of relieving stress. Read through the exercise to familiarize yourself with its steps, and then read through it a second time or have someone read it to you while you follow along to help your body relax. If you have a busy mind, you may have to do this exercise several times before you are able to focus on the physical aspects of the exercise without being distracted by your thoughts. Most people find that this exercise reduces tension but does not eliminate it altogether. Set a reasonable goal to reduce your tension a little bit each time you use the exercise. For example, if you rated your tension on a scale from 0 to 100, 100 would indicate total anxiety like the kind you may have experienced during a panic attack and a rating of 0 tension would occur only when you are in a deep sleep. If you start Exercise 15.6 at a tension level of 80, set a goal to reduce that tension to 65. If you set a goal that is too high, you will be disappointed and give up on the exercise. Because relaxation is a coping skill, you will get better with each practice.

Personal Resources: Use Your Strengths

In Exercise 5.3 in Chapter 5 you made a few notes about your coping resources. As you have been working through the exercises in this book, you have been developing new skills, and you have probably become more aware of coping abilities you already possessed. There are many ways that you can use your coping resources to deal with stress.

Many of the skills described in this book have focused on how to respond to stressful situations after they have occurred. You can use the same skills to deal with day-to-day experiences so that the accumulation of stress can be avoided. For example, if you lost your job but have avoided filing for unemployment benefits, your stress would climb as you ran out of money. You might have avoided filing because you had worries about the process, you didn't know if you could figure out how to file, you thought that filing for benefits would make you look like a loser, or it was difficult for you to get going in the morning because of depression. That happened to Joe. The longer he avoided it, the worse things got.

Joe has several coping resources available to him. He has people who can help him, such

EXERCISE 15.6 Relaxation Exercise

Find a comfortable and quiet place to sit or lie down. Take off your shoes, loosen your belt, take your hair out of your ponytail, or otherwise remove items that bind you too tightly. Keep a light on so you can read these instructions. **Take one deep breath** in through your nose and let it out through your mouth. As you do this, tell your body to let go of the tensions from head to toe. Continue to breathe normally and focus on releasing tensions from specific parts of your body. Let's **begin with your face**. Focus on relaxing your forehead. Smooth out any wrinkles, make your eyebrows relax, and think of tension dripping off your forehead and away from your body the way that sweat might drip off your forehead. Take a moment to loosen your forehead before going on.

When you're ready, turn your focus to your jaw and loosen it as much as you can. Loosen your jaw by letting your teeth part just a little. Release any tension you hold in your lips. Make sure your forehead stays relaxed and your jaw loose.

While keeping your eyes open enough to be able to read, try to relax your eyes. Feel tension leaving your face, falling away from your forehead, away from your eyes, and being released from your jaw. Your face is smoother, calmer, and more relaxed. Keep your face loose while you turn your attention to your shoulders and neck.

To begin to relax your **shoulders and neck,** let your shoulders drop and let your arms drop to your sides. Let the tension flow down your neck, down your shoulders, and away from your body. Picture your shoulder muscle being tight like a wet dishrag that you are wringing. Let your shoulders loosen just as you untwist the dishrag and shake it loose. Let the tension leave your neck and shoulders as you relax.

Let your attention go back to your face, search out any tightness you may have left there, and release it once again.

Next, it's time to allow your **arms** to relax. Starting at the top of your shoulders, allow the tension to leave those muscles. Feel your arms relax as you let them fall to your side. Relax your hands, let your fingers spread apart, and imagine tension flowing away from your body, down your arms, off your fingertips, and away from your body. Let your tensions melt away and drip off your fingertips and onto the floor like ice melting slowing.

Once again, focus on any remaining tension in your shoulders, allowing them to loosen further. Let relaxation flow through your face and neck, down your arms, and into your hands and fingers.

Now it's time to relax your **chest and stomach**. Continue to breathe normally, but as you exhale, focus on letting tension leave your body just as the air leaves your lungs. Feel relaxation spreading through your chest and stomach as you exhale. Take as long as you need to exhale away the tensions and breathe a sense of relaxation into your body.

Focus now on your stomach and allow it to relax. Release your stomach muscles, allowing them to loosen and feel more comfortable. Feel your body become more relaxed from your head to your shoulders, to your chest and throughout your stomach. Search out any tensions that remain and let them go free.

Now turn your attention to your **legs**. Uncross your legs or ankles if you have them crossed. Let the muscles relax throughout your legs and feet and all the way down to your toes. Loosen your toes, relax your ankles, and let your legs lie comfortably and relaxed. Imagine tension flowing down your legs, off your feet, and onto the floor.

Now **count from one to ten**, but as you say each number to yourself, try to relax just a little bit more. Let yourself focus on each group of muscles from head to toe, and when you find tension remaining, allow it to flow away from your body. **One**, focus on your face, letting go of any tension you find. **Two**, continue to let your shoulders drop and feel the tension flowing away from your neck and shoulders. **Three**, search your arms and hands and fingers. Allow them to continue to relax. **Four**, exhale, breathing out any remaining tensions in your chest. **Five**, loosen your stomach just a little bit more. **Six**, relax your right leg just a little bit more. Let it lie comfortably and loosely. **Seven**, turn your attention to your left leg. Allow it to loosen just a little bit more. **Eight**, once again scan your body from head to toe, find any remaining tensions in your muscles, and allow them to flow away from your body. **Nine**, as you exhale, notice that you're breathing more slowly and comfortably as you've allowed your body to slow down, to release the strains of the day, and to relax. **Ten**, enjoy the moment.

Memorize this feeling of relaxation. Notice how it is different from when you started this exercise. Tell your muscles to remember the sensation of relaxation so that you can go there again when you need to. Notice that your thoughts have slowed down. They are now easier to catch and focus on the things that are most important to you at this moment. When you're ready, allow yourself to pick a goal or a thought that needs your attention. Focus your energy on that single idea and see it to its conclusion.

as friends, family members, and his wife. He usually has a positive attitude about work once he sets his mind on a goal. He values financial responsibility. All of these things are resources that can help Joe take the necessary steps toward filing for unemployment benefits and finding another job. What are your coping resources?

Individual Coping Resources

When people are feeling bad, they often think they have nothing to offer the world. You read about this kind of thinking in Chapters 7, 10, and 11. A negative outlook can block from view your strengths, skills, abilities, and coping resources. If you use the exercises for correcting distorted thoughts, you may be able to reacquaint yourself with your strengths. You described some of these in the Chapter 3 exercises where you listed characteristics of the real you.

Your coping resources are the things within you and in your world that help you solve problems, deal with stress, and get things done. They can be physical things, like being strong, or they can be mental things, like being able to organize your time. Coping resources can include doing activities that give you hope, like going to your house of worship or being able to work or take care of your kids when you are tired. Internal fortitude, persistence, patience, a sense of humor, your faith in God, and your intelligence are all examples of your personal coping resources. You have them with you all the time, but sometimes they are hard to access or to remember. Sometimes you are unaware of your coping resources until you have a crisis to deal with and you see yourself in action.

What do you do when you absolutely have to do something and you don't feel up to it? Which of your coping resources do you use? Amanda provided a simple example. She agreed to bake a cake for an event at work, but her baking pans were in a high cupboard and she had left her stepladder at a church event. Amanda is short. What could she do? She had been feeling depressed, so she didn't really want to do anything. She didn't want to drive to the church to get her stepladder. She didn't want to ask for help. She didn't really want to bake the cake in the first place, but she also didn't want to show up at work empty-handed. She used Exercise 15.7 on the facing page to think about ways to cope with her dilemma.

Social Resources

People can be resources. They can be fountains of information, make suggestions for solving problems, give you advice, tell you how to do things differently, and take care of problems for you. While these can be good things, they are not always welcome when you are feeling bad. Mood swings can make you irritable and impatient with others. When they tell you things you already know, you might hear it as nagging. Their advice can seem naive if you think they truly do not understand your situation.

On the other hand, they may be right and their advice, if followed, might be helpful. Some "know-it-alls" actually know quite a bit that can be helpful. If you push away all advice when you are feeling bad, you might be missing out on a useful coping resource. When someone who cares about you gives you advice, use the exercises in Chapter 7 to keep negative emotions from controlling your thinking.

The coping assistance provided by people can take the form of emotional support even when no specific advice or assistance is given. A hug, a warm handshake, a smile of encouragement, or a nonjudgmental ear may not solve your problems, but they may give you the support you need to keep trying. Take a minute to complete Exercise 15.8 (p. 205) by listing the people in your world who are coping resources and what they do for you that seems helpful.

EXERCISE 15.7   What Are Your Coping Resources?

Think about a time you had to dig in and get something done. How did you force yourself to do it? What coping resources did you use? In the space provided, write down a current problem you are facing, and answer the questions below to help you identify your coping resources.

The problem is:

WHO? Who can help you cope when you are having trouble doing things on your own?

WHAT? What do you usually do when you absolutely must get something done even when you are not feeling up to it? What can you do to cope now?

WHERE? Where can you go for help if you are having trouble coping?

WHEN? When is it easiest for you to cope when you are not feeling your best? Are you a morning person, or do you do your best work at night?

HOW? How can you make yourself cope when you are feeling stressed?

Treatment Resources: Doctors, Therapists, Medications

Health care providers are obvious coping resources. They provide information, prescribe medications, teach coping skills, and offer a safe place to express your feelings without the risk of criticism. There are other ways that health care providers are coping resources. They help by adding structure to your life through regular appointments. They give you hope because they can see solutions when you are feeling overwhelmed. They understand you when your family doesn't. They show that they believe in you by having high expectations of you and by holding you accountable to do your best to control your symptoms. Clinicians take you seriously when others in your world might not. When times are tough, you can count on them for support. They don't give up on you, and they always want the best for you.

Like any other coping resource, health care providers will do you no good unless you use them. Mood swings can color your thinking and make you conclude that your health care provider doesn't care. Prepare for your next mood swing by making a few notes in Exercise 15.8 about how your health care providers have been helpful to you. Think about how feeling bad can keep you from asking for help when you need it the most and make a note in Exercise 15.9 on the facing page about what you should do the next time this happens.

AMANDA'S EXAMPLE **What Are Your Coping Resources?**

Think about a time you had to dig in and get something done. How did you force yourself to do it? What coping resources did you use? In the space provided, write down a current problem you are facing, and answer the questions below to help you identify your coping resources.

The problem is: *I have to bake a cake for work, and I can't reach the cake pans in the high cupboard.*

WHO? Who can help you cope when you are having trouble doing things on your own?
I can borrow a stepladder from my neighbor.
I can wait until someone comes home to help me reach the cake pans.

WHAT? What do you usually do when you absolutely must get something done even when you are not feeling up to it? What can you do to cope now?
I tell myself that I have to do it. I make a deal with myself for a small reward if I get the job done. I can always buy a cake on the way to work tomorrow even though I promised to make one.

WHERE? Where can you go for help if you are having trouble coping?
I can always go get a cake from somewhere like the grocery store. If I really need to bake, I can go to a friend's house to do it.

WHEN? When is it easiest for you to cope when you are not feeling your best? Are you a morning person, or do you do your best work at night?
I do best in the mornings. I run out of steam in the evenings. I will wait and bake the cake before work tomorrow. I don't mind getting up early. The house is quiet, and I can get someone to pull down the cake pans for me later tonight.

HOW? How can you make yourself cope when you are feeling stressed?
I will set an alarm.
I will prepare things tonight so I don't have to do much tomorrow.

EXERCISE 15.8 **People Who Help You Cope**

In the space below, list people you would consider coping resources. Make a note of what they do that is helpful. Some examples have been provided.

People who help you cope	What they do that is helpful
My grandmother *The guys at work*	*Tells me she loves me when I am feeling low.* *They have funny stories that make me laugh and forget about my problems for a while.*

EXERCISE 15.9 **What Should I Do Instead of Rejecting Help?**

In the space below, make a note to yourself about what you should do the next time you need help but don't want to ask for it. Tell yourself how to handle it.

AMANDA'S EXAMPLE What Should I Do Instead of Rejecting Help?

When I get depressed, I don't want to talk to anyone, especially my therapist and psychiatrist. I know what they will say, and I don't want to hear it. So I tough it out on my own and make my own adjustments to medications. Eventually, my family insists that I see the doctor because I am not getting any better. For the next mood swing, this is what I would like to say to myself:

You always think you know more than your doctor and therapist. You may know more, but when you are sick you don't make good decisions. You can't be objective. You need someone who can see more clearly than you. You don't have to like seeing your therapist; you just need to go see her. It is OK if your doctor is not as smart as you are; you still need help. Stop making excuses and use your resources.

What's Next?

This chapter was different from the previous ones in that it focused on strengthening your coping skills instead of trying to solve a problem or fix a symptom that has already emerged. During times when your mood is stable, you can use the exercises in this book to build your coping abilities. This will put you in a better position to cope when the next mood swing occurs.

The next chapter is similar in that it helps you build your ability to make good decisions. The methods can be used during times when your mood symptoms interfere with decision making and when you are feeling fine but facing a tough decision. Once you have mastered the new skills, return to this chapter and add better decision-making skills to your list of coping resources.

16

Make Better Decisions

In this chapter you will:

- ✓ Find new ways to stop avoiding important decisions.
- ✓ Learn the step-by-step approach to making decisions.

One way decision making can become impaired is that you can't organize your thoughts well enough to define the problem clearly or to consider all your options. Another possibility is that self-doubt creeps in and you become afraid that you'll make a bad decision. You reason to yourself that making no decision is better than making a bad decision and suffering the consequences. Sometimes decision making is a problem because the negative and hopeless thinking that accompanies depression makes every alternative seem unreasonable or untenable. Many times there are multiple problems that you are facing at the same time, and you are looking for a solution that can resolve several issues at a time and make the pieces of your life fall into place. This is more a fantasy than a reality because it is rare that you can solve all your problems with one intervention. Looking for the "right answer" or the "best choice" may keep you from choosing and implementing a solution. If you find that this is becoming a pattern with you, then you probably have this symptom.

Making Decisions

When you're making a choice between two options and one option stands out as better than the other, making a decision is easy. It gets more difficult when there are two or three less-than-perfect options and each has some definite advantages as well as some definite disadvantages.

Paul and his girlfriend have been together for 3 years. She has hinted around about marriage for the last 6 months. Angie is 2 years older than Paul and is ready to move on to the next stage of life. She wants to get married, buy a house, and have children. Angie loves Paul, but she thinks that he may be too immature to make this kind of commitment. She doesn't want to wait any longer, so she has asked Paul to marry her or let her go.

Paul loves Angie and doesn't want to lose her. She has stood by him as he has learned to control his illness and is tolerant of his "quirks." However, he is not sure he's ready for marriage. He has not established his career, and he may not be ready for the responsibilities of marriage, parenthood, and home ownership. Paul has to make a decision, and neither option, marriage or losing Angie, seemed like a good choice.

An even more complicated scenario arises when each choice has a clear advantage, but the advantages are very different. Let's say you're choosing a place to live and you find two possibilities for about the same price. One has more space, and the other has a better location. Which do you choose? Or what if you're choosing a college to go to and you're accepted by two, one where your closest friends are going and another that has a course of study you want to pursue? Which do you choose? If your thinking is clouded by emotion, overcrowded with racing thoughts, or slow and difficult to organize, you will have even more trouble making a decision. If you're like most people, you will put it off until you absolutely have to decide. Sometimes people will put off difficult decisions until the choice is made for them. For example, if Paul does not make a decision about marrying Angie, she will eventually leave him.

If you want to be more active in making decisions, you can follow the steps below for Exercise 16.1 on page 210. They will help you to sort out your options and choose the one that best meets your current needs. If you're not confident in your ability to reason through the choices, ask someone you trust for his or her opinion after you've completed the exercise. You may download and print additional copies of the Decision-Making Worksheet from *www.guilford.com/basco2-forms* and add them to your workbook as needed.

• **Step 1:** List the options you are weighing in the left-hand column of Exercise 16.1, the Decision-Making Worksheet. Work choices might include "*I can change jobs,*" "*I can remain at the existing job,*" and "*I can apply for Social Security disability and stop working.*" If you're trying to make a decision to end a relationship, the choices might include "*End it now,*" "*Stick it out longer and hope it gets better,*" and "*Tell my partner that I'm unhappy and ask if he [or she] is willing to work to make things better.*"

• **Step 2:** List the advantages and disadvantages of each choice. Some might overlap. For example, the advantages of staying at the same job (e.g., it is familiar and comfortable) might be the same as the disadvantages of changing jobs (e.g., it would put you in a new and possibly scary situation). Overlap is OK. List every advantage and disadvantage you can think of. Ask a friend or a family member to help you think of other pros and cons to each choice.

• **Step 3:** Read through the lists and pick out one or two of the strongest advantages and disadvantages of each decision choice. Circle these items. If it would be easier to read, you can cross off the others on your list.

- **Step 4:** Look for common themes in the advantages and disadvantages you listed. For example, if you're weighing the advantages and disadvantages of ending a relationship or staying with it, do you see *loneliness* versus *having someone to be with* as an issue? If so, it tells you that being with someone, not necessarily the person you are with now, is important to you. If you see stress reduction showing up as an advantage of making a change in jobs as well as a disadvantage of staying in your current job, then you know that your stress level is an important issue in your decisions. If you are trying to decide whether or not to change doctors, you might find the theme of familiarity and hating change in your advantages and disadvantages.

Examine the main advantages and disadvantages that you circled in Step 3 and try to pick out the main themes. List them on the Decision-Making Worksheet under "Themes."

- **Step 5:** To the right of each, rank-order the themes/issues according to their importance in making your decision. Make #1 the most important theme, #2 the second most important theme, and so on.

- **Step 6:** Once you have picked out the most important themes that will guide your decision making on a given problem and have arranged them in order of importance, it's time to match the themes to each of the decision options. This means going back to your original list of decision choices and picking out the ones that best match each theme. For example, if loneliness was the most important theme in making a decision about a relationship, pick the decision choice from your list of possible options that would be best for reducing your loneliness. If the second theme you identified was concern about money, go back to the list of decision choices and pick the one that best addresses your concern about money. To help you keep track, write each decision choice number from the Decision-Making Worksheet next to every theme that it matches.

- **Step 7:** Now that you have a list of themes and the decision choices that best match each theme, you can compare the items and choose the decision that addresses your issues best. You will know which it is by the number of themes each decision choice addresses. So if the decision choice you labeled as option 1 on the Decision-Making Worksheet does a good job of addressing each of the themes you identified, it's probably the best choice. If another decision choice addressed only one of your themes, and it was not the most important theme, it's probably not a good choice. The best options are those decision choices that address the most themes or issues or that at least address the most important themes.

You Don't Have to Do It Alone

Paul decided to share this worksheet with Angie (see p. 211) and asked her to fill one out too. If she was willing to wait, he was willing to commit to marriage. He needed time to prepare himself. He would work with his therapist on his emotional readiness and ask Angie to join them for some of their sessions. If Angie was not willing to wait, there was nothing he could do.

EXERCISE 16.1	Decision-Making Worksheet	
Possible options	**Advantages**	**Disadvantages**
Option 1:		
Option 2:		
Option 3:		

Themes	**Order of importance**	**Best options**

PAUL'S EXAMPLE Decision-Making Worksheet

Possible options	Advantages	Disadvantages
Option 1: Marry Angie	I get to keep her forever. She'll be happy and won't leave me. We can start working on building the lives we want.	I'm too young. I'll give up my independence. I won't have my parents to back me up financially. Marriage means more debt. Being together 24/7
Option 2: Break up with Angie	I will be able to finish my education without having to worry about money. I can date other people. I can hang out with my friends whenever I want. I don't have to burden Angie with my mood swings.	I will miss her terribly. I will never find anyone like her again. No one else will want to deal with my moodiness. I have to give up my dream of life and children with her. I will get severely depressed.
Option 3: Find a way to postpone marriage	I can keep Angie. I can take time to finish school and save some money. I can get ready to be a husband.	Angie says that she will not wait. If I postpone it too long, she will give up on me. She will start to hate me for making her put off her plans.

Themes	Order of importance	Best options
Losing Angie	1	1
Money	3	2 ③
Having someone who can understand me	2	1 ③
Being emotionally ready	4	2 ③

Here is another example.

Tommy had to move back in with his parents after his last hospitalization. He had been living with them for 9 months and thought he was ready to be on his own. His parents had paid for his apartments in the past, but he had always had to move back home either because he got evicted for excessive noise or for not keeping the place clean or because he was too ill to live on his own. Tommy's parents were not willing to go through that again, so they told him that if he wanted to live on his own he would have to pay for his own apartment. Tommy could not decide what to do, so he filled out a decision-making worksheet to help him sort through the issues. The choices he was considering were moving out on his own, getting a roommate, and continuing to stay with his parents for a while.

After he had worked through the exercise (see below), it became clear to Tommy that his best option would be to find a roommate and move out on his own. This choice addressed the issues or themes he had identified better than the other two options. He had a friend who lived in a one-bedroom apartment in the same city and was willing to rent a bigger apartment with Tommy and share expenses.

TOMMY'S EXAMPLE Decision-Making Worksheet

Possible options	Advantages	Disadvantages
Option 1: Move out on my own	Independence No one to stress me out Peace and quiet	Costs more money Loneliness Not sure I can handle it
Option 2: Get a roommate	Share expenses Might be fun Don't have to be alone	We might not get along. Limits my privacy We might have different habits.
Option 3: Live with my mom and dad	Save money for the future Have my own room Never lonely	No privacy Mom tells me what to do. Can't have people over

Themes	Order of importance	Best options
Independence, being on my own, and privacy	2	1, 2
Money	1	2, 3
Loneliness versus having someone around to talk to	3	2, 3

Getting Feedback from Others

You may not want to admit it, but sometimes other people who know you are right about what you should or should not do. They may be able to help you sort through your many ideas, decisions, choices, urges, and worries. Other people can be a resource if you let them. They may not always be right, but they can offer ideas that are different than yours and therefore challenge you to consider other possibilities.

When you are manic or hypomanic, you may have a lot more thoughts to sort through than usual. You also run the risk of making mistakes in logic and making poor choices because you've overlooked important facts. Most people regret making bad decisions when they are manic and want to learn methods for stopping themselves the next time before they act. The kinds of ideas that should alert you to be cautious are urges to make big changes in your life, to do something impulsive that would shock or surprise others, and to take risks that you would not normally take. When these ideas run through your mind, one strategy for protecting yourself is to tell someone about it. Even if you don't want the person's opinion or couldn't care less about his or her reaction, hearing yourself say the idea out loud can be enough to make you think it through before you act impulsively and regret it later.

Some people who have bipolar disorder don't feel comfortable verbalizing their impulsive thoughts because it makes other people overreact, become suspicious, watch them too closely, or behave in other negative ways toward them. These are valid concerns. No one wants to have a great idea shot down. On the other hand, to keep yourself out of trouble, you may need someone to help you apply the brakes. Identify a person in your world whom you can talk to about your ideas that others might find outrageous. Make sure it's someone who knows that just because you're thinking about taking risks doesn't mean you will actually do it. A therapist or psychiatrist can be that person, but it may be more practical to choose a family member, a friend, or someone else you know who has bipolar disorder and deals with similar thoughts from time to time. If you share your idea and get a negative reaction, apply the 24-hour rule.

Use Your Logic to Avoid Minimizing the Negatives

When entering a manic phase, you're susceptible to minimizing negatives. For example, you might overlook important details such as risks or disadvantages of situations. When you minimize negatives, the positive aspects of any idea can seem even more outstanding. You can convince yourself that there is no downside or that the risks are small and the benefits great even if this is not true.

To avoid minimizing, ask yourself and others the following questions:

- "What is the downside to my idea or plan?"
- "Are any risks involved?"

- "Could I be overlooking something important?"
- "Am I disregarding or ignoring important facts?"

Make yourself look at all the angles before drawing your conclusions and taking action. If Paul were going to use this strategy to sort out his thoughts about the new reading program he was inventing, he would answer these questions as follows:

- **"What is the downside to my idea or plan?"** *It will take a lot of time to work out the details of the program, and it may interfere with my other goals or with my sleep.*
- **"Are any risks involved?"** *If I put money into this plan, I could lose it if the idea is a flop. If I keep staying up late at night to work on it, I will probably get manic. I don't want to get manic again.*
- **"Could I be overlooking something important?"** *This could be just another of my manic fantasies that turns out to be a bad idea. I've been through times like this before.*
- **"Am I disregarding or ignoring important facts?"** *I don't know much about helping kids to read other than my own personal experience. I'm not sure what facts I'm overlooking.*

Gaining Emotional Distance

Paul gains emotional distance from his manic ideas by talking them over with his friends. For example, Paul talked to his friends at work about his reading program idea. After hearing their input he was not as convinced that it was the most wonderful idea he had ever had and that it was guaranteed to succeed. In fact, the more he talked to them about it, the less enthusiastic Paul felt about working on the idea. Knowing himself and his tendency to get caught up in his own fantasies, he dismissed the idea as a manic thought and focused on his current work responsibilities.

Making the Decision to Take Care of Yourself

If taking precautions by keeping a more consistent sleep schedule, monitoring your symptoms, and limiting overstimulation sounds like too much restriction on your lifestyle, you may not want to do it. You certainly have the right to do as you please, take the risks you want, and deal with any consequences that may follow. It's your decision to follow or not follow the guidelines in this workbook, to take the advice of your therapist, or to take medication the way your psychiatrist tells you to. If you live alone and do not have responsibilities to others, you will be the only one to suffer the costs of not taking precautions. It may not be a big deal. But if other people depend on you and a return of your depression or mania will affect their lives, your decision should probably take them into consideration.

Be sure not to view taking precautions in an all-or-nothing way. It's not a matter of total restriction versus total freedom. You may be able to make some changes in your routine to better suit your illness or try to take precautions as often as possible, knowing there will be times when your lifestyle will not allow it. Also, consider the possibility that you may not be ready to make the kinds of changes in your routine that are being recommended by the workbook, your family, or your health care providers. That doesn't mean you won't be more ready next month or next year or the next time you have symptoms. Taking care of yourself will always be a good idea no matter when you start taking the right action. If you know you can't do it right now, put this book back on your shelf and look it over again later. Life circumstances can change quickly and create new opportunities for you to take control of your symptoms.

What's Next?

You probably have no difficulty making decisions most of the time, especially when you are feeling well. Symptoms of depression and mania, however, can make it difficult to think through and resolve problems. The purpose of this chapter was to provide you with exercises that can help you make decisions at times when you are feeling stuck. Learning to systematically weigh the pros and cons of your life choices can help you when your mood swings interfere with your creativity, leave you with self-doubt, or make it hard for you to concentrate. In the next chapter, you will have a chance to make some decisions about how to maintain the gains you have achieved as you have worked through this book. Use this opportunity to think about all that you have learned and set some goals for maintaining your gains.

17

Maintain Your Gains

In this chapter you will:

✓ Learn how to evaluate your progress.

✓ Make a plan for continued self-improvement.

✓ Check on your acceptance of your mood swings.

Stay Self-Aware

To be able to control your mood swings you have to become tuned in to the subtle variations in your feelings, thoughts, and actions that signal a change. Many of the exercises in this workbook were designed to help you become more self-aware. Not everyone has the ability to notice their mood changes even when they are obvious to others. To successfully control your symptoms, you may have to rely on others to alert you that your mood is changing. While this kind of feedback can be very helpful, it can also create problems in your relationships, especially when the person giving you feedback is wrong. In some relationships, the person with the mood swings is scapegoated by being blamed for problems he or she did not create.

Check Your Progress

The exercises provided throughout this workbook have encouraged you to be specific about your goals and your plans. Now that you've read through the various methods for controlling your symptoms of depression and mania, make a few notes in Exercise 17.1 on page 218 about the steps you have already taken or plan to take to accomplish each of these aims.

The goals emphasized throughout this workbook are:

- to **know yourself**, your vulnerabilities, your strengths, and your symptoms well
- to **practice** and strengthen the skills for managing your illness that have been described in this workbook
- to **learn from each episode** of illness you experience so that you know what to watch for next time
- to **work toward acceptance** of having bipolar disorder so that you can move forward, do everything you can to stay well, and get on with your life
- to **avoid risks** of relapse
- to **find a medication** regimen you feel comfortable enough to follow

Many people will master the techniques in this workbook but find that their symptoms return anyway. Because bipolar disorder is a recurring illness, you should count on there being times when your symptoms return. There are a few lucky people who find exactly the right medication, take it religiously, and never have mania or depression again. Unfortunately, they are not in the majority. The goal of managing bipolar disorder is to decrease the number of episodes of depression and mania as much as possible, eliminate the milder symptoms that can continue between episodes, and, if a relapse does occur, catch and contain it as quickly as possible. This way you will spend more time feeling well and less time feeling ill as you learn more and more about controlling the illness.

Monitor Your Mood

The methods you learned in Chapter 4 for recognizing symptoms of depression and mania and for monitoring daily mood changes can help you check on your progress. If you were rating yourself regularly on a Mood Graph (see Exercise 17.2 on p. 219), what you would hope to see is a steady improvement in your mood over time and then more stability in your mood. This means that if you rated your mood each day and connected the dots on the graph, you would see a line through the middle with fluctuations between −1 and +1 most of the time. When your mood dropped toward depression or climbed toward mania, you would hope to see those changes return to normal within a few days. And if you use the new tools you have learned in this workbook as often as possible, you should have fewer and fewer days with ratings above +2 or below −2.

If you decide not to keep Mood Graphs on a daily basis, you can use them periodically to check on how you're doing. For example, if you know you tend to get depressed in the winter and manic during the spring, you might start keeping a Mood Graph just before those seasons begin. If you see that your graph is moving toward more symptoms, use the methods you've learned to stop their progression and contact your doctor when you see that the daily ratings are not improving or the symptoms are becoming more difficult to manage on your own. When the season is over, keep a Mood Graph for another week or two to be certain

Ways I have gotten to know my vulnerabilities, my strengths, and my symptoms better. My plan for learning more about myself and my illness.

My thoughts on how to practice and strengthen my skills for managing my illness that have been described in this workbook.

How I might learn from each episode of illness I experience so that I know what to watch for next time.

What I need to do to work toward acceptance of having bipolar disorder so that I can move forward, do everything I can to stay well, and get on with my life.

Things I know I can do to avoid the risk of relapse.

How I will find a medication regimen I feel comfortable enough to follow.

Mood Graph

Use this worksheet to track your mood each day.								
Week of:	**Plan**	**Sun**	**Mon**	**Tues**	**Wed**	**Thur**	**Fri**	**Sat**
Manic **+5** Not sleeping, psychotic	*Go to the hospital*	●	●	●	●	●	●	●
+4 Manic, poor judgment		●	●	●	●	●	●	●
+3 Hypomanic	*Call the doctor*	●	●	●	●	●	●	●
+2 Energized	*Take action*	●	●	●	●	●	●	●
+1 Hyper, happy	*Watch closely*	●	●	●	●	●	●	●
0 Normal		●	●	●	●	●	●	●
−1 Low, down	*Watch closely*	●	●	●	●	●	●	●
−2 Sad	*Take action*	●	●	●	●	●	●	●
−3 Depressed	*Call the doctor*	●	●	●	●	●	●	●
−4 Immobilized		●	●	●	●	●	●	●
−5 Suicidal **Depressed**	*Go to the hospital*	●	●	●	●	●	●	●

What caused the mood shift?

that your mood is remaining stable. You may download and print extra copies of the Mood Graph form from *www.guilford.com/basco2-forms.*

Adjustment and Acceptance

If you've struggled with acceptance of having bipolar disorder, your efforts throughout this workbook may have helped you progress through the stages of adjustment. Review the thoughts and behaviors associated with each stage of adjustment in Exercise 17.3 on the facing page to see if you can recognize where you are today. Compare your answers to those you marked on Exercise 12.1 in Chapter 12 (p. 160).

Goal Setting

It is pretty common practice to set goals. People do it all the time. Setting goals can provide you with direction, and it can be motivating to write down the things you would like to accomplish. Completing tasks and crossing them off your to-do list can leave you with a sense of accomplishment even when the accomplishments are small. Unfortunately, mood swings can make it difficult to set and complete our goals. For example, when you feel yourself getting overstimulated or overwhelmed by too many ideas or too much to do, you might find yourself going in too many directions at one time. The Goal-Setting Worksheet in Exercise 17.4 (p. 222) can help you organize your thoughts when mania and hypomania begin to emerge. You may download and print additional copies of the Goal-Setting Worksheet from *www.guilford.com/basco2-forms* and add them to your workbook as needed.

Use the Goal-Setting Worksheet to write down all the activity ideas that come to mind. This would include things you have to do, things you want to do, and things you've been putting off for some time. Once you have them all written down, try to determine whether each item is a high (H), medium (M), or low (L) priority. There is a column with **H**, **M**, and **L** next to each item. Circle the one that applies. *High priority* can mean that the task is something very important or has an immediate deadline. High-priority tasks might include paying your rent or getting your medication refilled. *Low-priority* tasks are those that can wait, like watching a particular movie or reorganizing your closet. There is no consequence if they don't get done right away. Low-priority tasks also include things that have only a small consequence if not completed; for example, going to the grocery store to buy more milk. You would like to do it if you had time, but it's not an emergency. *Medium-priority* tasks are somewhere in the middle between high- and low-priority tasks.

When you are finished with your list and have made your priority ratings, review the list. If you have too many items marked as high priorities, reconsider whether these are things that absolutely must be done right away or could wait until you have more time. On the first pass, it's easy to think that everything is a high priority even when it is not.

For the items that really are high priorities, put them in order of how you want to

EXERCISE 17.3	Stages of Adjustment	
Stage	**Automatic thoughts**	**Actions**
Denial	• *I don't have it. The doctor made a mistake.* • *It must be because I've been drinking too much.* • *The diagnosis is wrong.*	• Getting a second opinion • Looking for other explanations for symptoms • Ignoring treatment recommendations
Anger	• *It's not fair that I have this illness.* • *I can't deal with this right now.* • *Why me? What did I do to deserve this?*	• Refusing to listen to advice • Refusing to discuss the illness • Losing temper with health care providers, pharmacies, or anyone else associated with treatment
Bargaining	• *I'll clean up my act.* • *I'll stop drinking, start waking up on time, start exercising, get a better job, and it will be OK.* • *I'll try natural remedies. I don't really need medicine.*	• Adjusting doses on your own • Changing the timing of doses • Trading active drugs for "natural remedies" • Staying up late to avoid taking sleeping medications • Drinking alcohol to reduce anxiety
Depression	• *I'll never have a normal life.* • *No one will want me.* • *I hate myself.*	• Self-destructive behaviors • Avoidance of stimuli related to the illness • Withdrawal from others
Acceptance	• *I can work my way through this.* • *It's not the end of the world.* • *I don't have to give up everything just because I have to take medication.*	• Adherence to treatment • Open discussion of treatment options with clinicians before discontinuing medications

Current activities, responsibilities, and interests	Priority			Rank order
	High	Medium	Low	
_____	H	M	L	____
_____	H	M	L	____
_____	H	M	L	____
_____	H	M	L	____
_____	H	M	L	____
_____	H	M	L	____
_____	H	M	L	____
_____	H	M	L	____
_____	H	M	L	____
_____	H	M	L	____
_____	H	M	L	____
_____	H	M	L	____
_____	H	M	L	____
_____	H	M	L	____
_____	H	M	L	____
_____	H	M	L	____
_____	H	M	L	____
_____	H	M	L	____
_____	H	M	L	____
_____	H	M	L	____

Goal-Setting Worksheet

| | Priority | | | Rank order |
Current activities, responsibilities, and interests	High	Medium	Low	
Finish reading new book	H	M	(L)	____
Pay the rent	(H)	M	L	1
Return Mom's call	H	(M)	L	____
Get oil changed in car	H	(M)	L	____
Ask Angie out for Friday night	(H)	M	L	2
Make a bank deposit	H	(M)	L	____
Figure out codes on PS4 game	H	M	(L)	____
Take in computer to be repaired	(H)	M	L	6
Buy groceries	H	(M)	L	____
Buy cigars	(H)	M	L	7
Refill med prescription	H	(M)	L	____
Do laundry—underwear	(H)	M	L	3
Go to work	(H)	M	L	5
Fix broken window on car	(H)	M	L	4
	H	M	L	____
	H	M	L	____
	H	M	L	____
	H	M	L	____
	H	M	L	____
	H	M	L	____

From *The Bipolar Workbook, Second Edition.* Copyright 2015 by The Guilford Press.

complete them, with *1* next to the most important and highest-priority item, *2* next to the second-most-important item, and so on. Put these numbers in the column labeled "Rank order."

Next comes the hard part. You have to make yourself do one thing at a time, starting with the highest-priority item. Even though your instinct may be to jump from one activity to another, make a deal with yourself to finish one task before going on to the next.

Planning Ahead to Accomplish Your Goals

In Chapter 13, behavioral contracts were introduced as a way of planning ahead for obstacles that might interfere with achieving your treatment goals. Take a moment and think about what could keep you from achieving the goals of this workbook and write them in Exercise 17.5 on the following page.

If you use the methods in this workbook, you'll find that with practice you will be able to:

Get the Big Picture

- Understand your mood swings and figure out what you can do to help yourself.
- Learn about the symptoms of bipolar disorder.
- Figure out the difference between a mood swing and the real you.

See It Coming

- See the changes coming—learn to recognize and label your moods.
- Know what triggers your mood swings and improve your coping.

Don't Make It Worse

- Avoid things that make your mood worse.
- Don't let emotions control your thinking.
- Stop avoidance and procrastination.

Reduce Your Symptoms

- Regain control when you feel overwhelmed.
- Change your negative outlook.
- Learn to analyze your thoughts.
- Work through denial about needing medication.
- Improve medication consistency.

Goal: Prevent recurrences of depression and mania

Potential obstacles to achieving this goal:

What I can do to overcome this obstacle:

Goal: Learn when my symptoms are returning

Potential obstacles to achieving this goal:

What I can do to overcome this obstacle:

Goal: Take action to control symptoms before they become full episodes of depression and mania

Potential obstacles to achieving this goal:

What I can do to overcome this obstacle:

Goal: Correct and control the thinking problems, activity changes, and emotional upsets caused by the illness

Potential obstacles to achieving this goal:

What I can do to overcome this obstacle:

Strengthen Your Coping Skills

- Learn to deal effectively with problems.
- Strengthen your stress management skills and healthy habits.
- Make better decisions.
- Maintain your gains.

Remember that each time you experience depression, mania, hypomania, or mixed states, you have an opportunity to put your new tools to the test, evaluate their precision, and refine them for times to come.

What's Next?

Now that you've learned the tools for controlling your symptoms of bipolar disorder, it's time to put them into practice. Controlling the symptoms of bipolar disorder is an ongoing process. This workbook was written to help you through that process. Refer back to the guidelines and exercises as you encounter symptoms or problems along the way. Even when times are good and you are feeling fine, review the strategies for staying well and for managing your lifestyle.

Share your work with your therapist or psychiatrist so that he or she will know what you're doing to manage your illness. Find a way to remind yourself from time to time to check on your symptoms and make the adjustments you've learned to keep them under control.

If you hit a rough spot and depression or mania returns, do your part to pull yourself together. Learn from the experience by analyzing what occurred that might have made you vulnerable to relapse. Each time you have symptoms and get them under control, you learn more about how to prevent them the next time.

Self-improvement is an ongoing process. It is normal to make gains, have setbacks, and have to start over again sometimes. Keep this workbook where you can use it as a reminder to practice the skills you have learned. Reread the sections that seem to fit you best. Pick the methods that work and practice them until they become part of your normal routine. Once you feel like you have mastered a skill, pick a new one to learn. The goal is to increase your skills for managing your mood swings. Make a commitment to yourself to do all that you can to help yourself. Good luck.

Resources

Books on Bipolar Disorder

Monica Ramirez Basco and A. John Rush. (2007). *Cognitive-Behavioral Therapy for Bipolar Disorder* (2nd ed.). New York: Guilford Press.

Thilo Deckersbach, Britta Hölzel, Lori Eisner, Sara W. Lazar, and Andrew A. Nierenberg. (2014). *Mindfulness-Based Cognitive Therapy for Bipolar Disorder*. New York: Guilford Press.

Jan Fawcett, Bernard Golden, and Nancy Rosenfeld. (2007). *New Hope for People with Bipolar Disorder: Your Friendly Authoritative Guide to the Latest in Traditional and Complementary Solutions* (2nd ed.). New York: Random House.

Mary A. Fristad, Jill S. Goldberg Arnold, and Jarrod M. Leffler. (2011). *Psychotherapy for Children with Bipolar and Depressive Disorders*. New York: Guilford Press.

Frederick K. Goodwin and Kay Redfield Jamison. (2007). *Manic Depressive Illness: Bipolar Disorders and Recurrent Depression* (2nd ed.). Oxford: Oxford University Press.

Kay Redfield Jamison. (1996). *Touched with Fire: Manic Depressive Illness and the Artistic Temperament*. New York: Simon & Schuster.

Cynthia G. Last. (2009). *When Someone You Love Is Bipolar: Help and Support for You and Your Partner*. New York: Guilford Press.

John McManamy. (2006). *Living Well with Depression and Bipolar Disorder: What Your Doctor Doesn't Tell You . . . That You Need to Know*. New York: HarperCollins.

David J. Miklowitz. (2011). *The Bipolar Disorder Survival Guide: What You and Your Family Need to Know* (2nd ed.). New York: Guilford Press.

David J. Miklowitz and Michael J. Gitlin. (2014). *Clinician's Guide to Bipolar Disorder: Integrating Pharmacology and Psychotherapy*. New York: Guilford Press.

Frances Mark Mondimore. (2014). *Bipolar Disorder: A Guide for Patients and Families*. Baltimore: Johns Hopkins University Press.

Mani Pavuluri. (2008). *What Works for Bipolar Kids: Help and Hope for Parents*. New York: Guilford Press.

Jesse H. Wright, David Kingdon, Douglas Turkington, and Monica Ramirez Basco. (2008). *Cognitive-Behavior Therapy for Severe Mental Illness*. Washington, DC: American Psychiatric Press.

Online Resources for Bipolar Disorder

American Psychiatric Association
www.psychiatry.org/bipolar-disorder

American Psychological Association
www.apa.org/topics/bipolar/index.aspx

Bipolar World
www.bipolarworld.net

BP Magazine
www.bphope.com

Depression and Bipolar Support Alliance
www.dbsalliance.org

McMan's Depression and Bipolar Web
www.mcmanweb.com

National Alliance on Mental Illness
www.nami.org

National Institute of Mental Health: Information on Bipolar Disorder
www.nimh.nih.gov
or
www.nimh.nih.gov/health/topics/bipolar-disorder/index.shtml

U.S. Department of Veterans Affairs
www.mentalhealth.va.gov/bipolar.asp

WebMD
www.webmd.com/bipolar-disorder/default.htm

Index

About the Author

Monica Ramirez Basco, PhD, is a clinical psychologist, author, and health scientist administrator at the National Institutes of Health. She currently serves as Assistant Director for Neuroscience, Mental Health, and Broadening Participation at the White House Office of Science and Technology Policy. Dr. Basco is an internationally recognized expert in cognitive-behavioral therapy and a founding fellow of the Academy of Cognitive Therapy.